www.harcourt-  com

Bringing you products from ...ences companies including Baillià ...igstone, Mosby and W.B. Saunders

- ◉ **Browse** for latest information on new books, journals and electronic products

- ◉ **Search** for information on over 20 000 published titles with full product information including tables of contents and sample chapters

- ◉ **Keep up to date** with our extensive publishing programme in your field by registering with eAlert or requesting postal updates

- ◉ **Secure online ordering** with prompt delivery, as well as full contact details to order by phone, fax or post

- ◉ **News** of special features and promotions

If you are based in the following countries, please visit the country-specific site to receive full details of product availability and local ordering information

USA: www.harcourthealth.com

Canada: www.harcourtcanada.com

Australia: www.harcourt.com.au

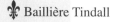 Baillière Tindall 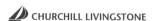 CHURCHILL LIVINGSTONE Mosby 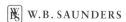 W.B. SAUNDERS

Postnatal Care

For Churchill Livingstone:

Commissioning Editor: Inta Ozols
Project Development Manager: Mairi McCubbin
Project Manager: Jane Dingwall
Designer: George Ajayi

Postnatal Care
Evidence and Guidelines for Management

Debra Bick BA MMedSci RGN RM
Senior Research and Development Fellow, Royal College of Nursing Institute, Oxford, UK; formerly Research Fellow in Midwifery, Department of Public Health and Epidemiology, University of Birmingham, Edgbaston, UK

Christine MacArthur PhD
Professor of Maternal and Child Epidemiology, Department of Public Health and Epidemiology, University of Birmingham, Edgbaston, UK

Helena Knowles BSc MPhil RGN RM
Academic Midwife Teacher, Institute of Health and Community Studies, Bournemouth University, UK; formerly Research Midwife, Department of Public Health and Epidemiology, University of Birmingham, Edgbaston, UK

Heather Winter MD FRCOG MFPHM
Senior Clinical Lecturer in Public Health and Epidemiology, Department of Public Health and Epidemiology, University of Birmingham, Edgbaston, UK

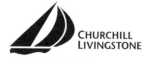

CHURCHILL LIVINGSTONE

EDINBURGH LONDON NEW YORK PHILADELPHIA ST LOUIS SYDNEY TORONTO 2002

CHURCHILL LIVINGSTONE
An imprint of Harcourt Publishers Limited

© Harcourt Publishers Limited 2002

 is a registered trademark of Harcourt Publishers Limited

The right of Debra Bick, Christine MacArthur, Helena Knowles and
Heather Winter to be identified as authors of this work has been
asserted by them in accordance with the Copyright, Designs and
Patents Act 1988

First published 2002

ISBN 0 443 064911

British Library Cataloguing in Publication Data
A catalogue record for this book is available from the British Library

Library of Congress Cataloging in Publication Data
A catalog record for this book is available from the Library of
Congress

Note
Medical knowledge is constantly changing. As new information
becomes available, changes in treatment, procedures, equipment and
the use of drugs become necessary. The authors and the publishers
have taken care to ensure that the information given in this text is
accurate and up to date. However, readers are strongly advised to
confirm that the information, especially with regard to drug usage,
complies with the latest legislation and standards of practice.

The
publisher's
policy is to use
**paper manufactured
from sustainabe forests**

Printed in China

Contents

Summary Guideline leaflets are repeated in the inside back pocket

Advisory group

The following members of the IMPaCT study team gave advice and comments to the authors at various stages of the drafting of the guidelines.

Ms Christine Henderson, Senior Research Fellow, School of Health Sciences, University of Birmingham.

Professor Richard Lilford, Professor of Clinical Epidemiology, Department of Public Health and Epidemiology, University of Birmingham, and Director of NHS Research and Development, NHS Executive West Midlands.

Mr Harry Gee, Senior Lecturer, Department of Obstetrics and Gynaecology, Birmingham Women's Health Care NHS Trust.

Christine Henderson devised the format of the accompanying leaflet sections of the guidelines.

ACKNOWLEDGEMENTS

The Guidelines were developed as part of a randomised controlled trial funded by the NHS R&D Health Technology Assessment Programme and we would like to acknowledge their support. We would like to thank the 80 midwives who took part in the trial, which allowed us to evaluate the use of the guidelines in community postnatal practice. Thanks also to Anne Walker who carefully prepared the drafts of the manuscript and Anne Fry-Smith from ARIF who assisted with the search strategies.

External peer reviewers

ENDOMETRITIS AND ABNORMAL BLOOD LOSS
Dr Sally Marchant RN RM ADM Diploma in Research Studies PhD
Senior Lecturer in Midwifery, Institute of Health and Community Studies,
Bournemouth University

PERINEAL PAIN AND DYSPAREUNIA
Mrs Christine Kettle SRN SCM DipMS
Midwifery Research Fellow, North Staffordshire Hospital Centre NHS Trust

Mr Richard Johanson MA BSc MBBChir MRCOG MD
Consultant Obstetrician/Senior Lecturer, North Staffordshire Hospital Centre
NHS Trust/Keele University

CAESAREAN SECTION WOUND CARE AND PAIN RELIEF
Mrs Pauline M Hobbs SRN BSc
Infection Control Nurse Specialist, Department of Microbiology,
Birmingham Women's Hospital NHS Trust

Dr Richard H George MBChB FRCPath
Consultant Microbiologist, Department of Microbiology,
Birmingham Women's Hospital NHS Trust

BREASTFEEDING ISSUES
Professor Mary Renfrew BSc RGN SCM RN (Canada) PhD
Professor of Midwifery Studies/Head of Division of Midwifery,
Mother and Infant Research Unit, University of Leeds

Mrs Christine Carson SRN SCM PGDip MSc
National Infant Feeding Adviser, Department of Health

URINARY PROBLEMS
Professor Linda Cardozo MD FRCOG
Professor of Urogynaecology, Department of Obstetrics,
King's College Hospital, London

Ms Nina Bridges SRP MCSP
Physiotherapy Manager, Department of Physiotherapy,
Birmingham Women's Hospital NHS Trust

BOWEL PROBLEMS
Professor Michael Keighley MS FRCS
Barling Professor of Surgery, Head of Department of Surgery,
University of Birmingham

Mr Abdul Sultan MBChB MRCOG MD
Consultant Obstetrician and Gynaecologist,
Mayday Hospital, Surrey

DEPRESSION AND OTHER PSYCHOLOGICAL MORBIDITY
Professor John Cox DM FRCPsych
Head of Department/Professor of Psychiatry,
Department of Psychiatry, University of Keele;
President, The Royal College of Psychiatrists, London

Mrs Gail Chapman RM MPhil
Research Midwife, Academic Department of Obstetrics and Gynaecology,
North Staffordshire Hospital NHS Trust

BACKACHE
Dr Martin Wilkinson MMedSci FRCGP
Lecturer, Department of Primary Care and General Practice,
University of Birmingham

Ms Ros Davies MCSP SRP
Senior Physiotherapist, Department of Physiotherapy,
Birmingham Women's Hospital NHS Trust

HEADACHE
Dr Griselda Cooper MB ChB FRCA
Senior Lecturer in Anaesthetics, University of Birmingham

Mr Andrew Shennan MBBS MRCOG MD
Senior Lecturer in Maternal and Fetal Health,
Fetal Health Research Group, King's College,
University of London

Preface

The evidence base and guidelines which form the main part of this book were developed as part of the IMPaCT (Implementing Midwifery-led Postnatal Care Trial) study. This was a randomised controlled trial testing a new model of midwifery-led postnatal care, the main objective of which was to improve women's physical and psychological health after birth, through the systematic identification and management of their postpartum health problems. These guidelines were part of the new care package used by the community midwives in the study to provide best evidence of effective management. As such they have been extensively reviewed and tested.

The guidelines were devised for use by practising midwives and assume a prior level of knowledge applicable to their training and experience, but may be useful for other groups, such as midwifery and nursing students, health visitors, general practitioners and obstetricians, as well as women themselves. Although prepared for UK postnatal practice, they are applicable to community based care after childbirth in other countries in the developed world.

The following pages give a brief background to the IMPaCT study and the role of the guidelines in this, followed by a description of the methods used to develop the guidelines. A section on how best to use the guidelines follows.

Background to the IMPaCT study

During the last decade, the UK maternity services were the focus of two major reports, the recommendations of which sought to influence the future direction of the services. In 1992, the House of Commons Health Committee report on the maternity services was published (House of Commons Health Committee 1992) which, among other findings, highlighted the neglect of postnatal care and lack of research in the area. This was followed by the establishment of the Expert Maternity Committee, whose remit was to examine policy and make recommendations for the maternity services in England and Wales. Their report *Changing childbirth* (Department of Health 1993) recommended that the maternity services should offer women more choice, greater continuity of care, more involvement in the planning of their care and should be a midwifery-led service. These reports coincided with data becoming available from studies in the UK and elsewhere systematically documenting significant postpartum physical and psychological health problems, many of which were not reported to or identified by the maternity services (Brown & Lumley 1998, Garcia & Marchant 1993, Glazener et al 1995, MacArthur et al 1991).

Responsibility in the UK for postnatal care after hospital discharge lies with the primary health care team. Midwives provide the majority of this care, but receive limited guidance on the content of this, despite a statutory obligation to attend women for a minimum of 10, up to a maximum of 28, days after delivery (UKCC 1998). Midwifery postnatal care has traditionally focused on routine examinations and observations until around the 10th day, when care is transferred to the health visitor. Until 1986 midwives were obliged to make daily home visits for the first 10 days, then the UKCC introduced a policy of 'selective' visiting, but with no evidence to support this change and no guidance on how to select visits. The other major change in UK practice, which has occurred more gradually, is the earlier discharge of women from hospital, with consequences for the workload of the community midwife, and making effective community postnatal care even more important.

In addition to midwife visits, many GPs make routine home visits and all women are offered a GP consultation at 6–8 weeks, marking the discharge from the routine maternity services. Although uptake of this consultation is high (Bick & MacArthur 1995, Bowers 1985) it appears to be based more on tradition than need, with abdominal and vaginal examinations routinely included, and has substantial NHS resource implications, without evidence of effect or appropriateness of timing (Noble 1993, Sharif & Jordan 1995, Sharif et al 1993).

Recent studies of maternal morbidity have consistently found that women will give information about their health problems *if they are asked*, but they often do not voluntarily report these to relevant health professionals (Bick & MacArthur 1995, Brown & Lumley 1998, Glazener et al 1995, MacArthur et al 1991). It was proposed that much morbidity remained unidentified because of the time-consuming focus of care on routine observations and examinations and the early discharge from maternity services, leaving insufficient opportunity to ascertain and manage women's health needs adequately.

With these unmet maternal health needs in mind and following the recommended changes to the UK maternity services, a team of researchers in the Department of Public Health and Epidemiology at the University of Birmingham designed and have carried out a randomised controlled trial of a new model of midwifery-led postnatal care (IMPaCT), funded by the NHS Research and Development Health Technology Assessment Programme. The new model of care enabled midwives to plan selective visits based on the individual needs of women until the twenty eighth rather than the tenth day. They used a symptom checklist to systematically identify physical and psychological health problems on about the tenth and twenty eighth days, then at the final discharge consultation. Replacing the GP 6–8 week postnatal check, this was undertaken by the midwives, and took place at 10–12 weeks, allowing women time after such a major life event to consider their own health needs (see Appendix 2). The Edinburgh Postnatal Depression Scale (EPDS) (Appendix 3) was also administered on day 28 and at the 10–12 week check, to identify women who were at risk of developing depression. The emphasis of the new model of care at all times was on the identification and appropriate management, including support and reassurance, of individual physical and psychological health needs. The evidence based guidelines were developed to help achieve this.

The findings on the outcomes of the trial will be published in due course in appropriate journals, but in the absence of any evidence based information for midwives and other professionals on the management of postnatal health problems, and following numerous requests nationally and internationally from groups and individuals to obtain copies, it was decided that the full set of guidelines should be made available.

Development of the guidelines

The procedure used to develop the guidelines was extensive and scientifically rigorous and took various stages, which are described briefly below and are detailed in Appendix 1.

1. A comprehensive search of the literature was undertaken by members of the team on health problems experienced by postnatal women, to ensure that the set of guidelines should encompass the whole range of these. The literature was then searched to obtain evidence on the management of each problem area, using recognised search strategies based on the 'hierarchy of evidence' and undertaken with assistance from experts (see Appendix 1).

These summaries of evidence are not formal systematic reviews. The scarcity of good quality research on postnatal care has been widely recognised and where available was often subject to methodological weaknesses. As an alternative to repeatedly stating this, where the quality of evidence was higher, this has been emphasised.

2. Using the above information, each guideline was then drafted by at least two of the authors.

3. The guidelines were then reviewed by other members of the study team, which included midwives, obstetricians, general practitioners and epidemiologists, and then revised.

4. One or more national experts in the various subject areas then reviewed the guidelines, which were revised following any comments.

5. A group of practising community midwives in another health region were given the full set of guidelines and asked for comments based on application to practice. Some further revisions were made.

6. The guidelines were then ready for use in the new model of care to be provided by the community midwives attached to the randomly selected general practices included in the IMPaCT study.

7. Following completion of their use in the study and informed by this, the guidelines were updated and amended by the authors, also taking account of any new evidence, and were reviewed again by the same national experts.

REFERENCES

Bick D E, MacArthur C 1995 Attendance, content and relevance of the six week postnatal examination. Midwifery 11: 69–73

Bowers J 1985 Is the 6 week postnatal examination necessary? The Practitioner. December 229: 1113–1115

Brown S, Lumley J 1998 Maternal health after childbirth: results of an Australian population based survey. Br J Obstet Gynaecol 105: 156–161

Department of Health 1993 Changing childbirth. The report of the Expert Maternity Group. HMSO, London

Garcia J, Marchant S 1993 Back to normal? Postpartum health and illness. In: Robinson S, Tickner V (eds) 1992 Research and the midwife. Conference proceedings 1992. University of Manchester

Glazener C M A, Abdalla M, Stroud P et al 1995 Postnatal maternal morbidity: extent, causes, prevention and treatment. Br J Obstet Gynaecol 102: 282–287

House of Commons Health Committee 1992 Report: Maternity services. HMSO, London, vol 1

MacArthur C, Lewis M, Knox E G 1991 Health after childbirth. HMSO, London

Noble T 1993 The routine six week postnatal vaginal examination. Forget it. BMJ 307: 698

Sharif K, Jordan J 1995 The six week postnatal visit – are we doing it right? Br J Hosp Med 54: 7–10

Sharif K, Clarke P, Whittle M 1993 Routine six week postnatal vaginal examination; to do or not to do? J Obstet Gynaecol 4(13): 151–152

United Kingdom Central Council for Midwifery and Health Visiting (UKCC) 1998 Midwives' rules and code of practice. UKCC, London

How to use the guidelines

FORMAT OF THE GUIDELINES

Each guideline has three sections as described below.

The **first section** presents the *full review of evidence* relating to each health problem or symptom, including definition, frequency of occurrence, risk factors and management. The evidence presented, although focused on primary management by the midwife, often includes information on GP primary management and sometimes includes evidence on secondary management, in order that a comprehensive picture is made available.

The **second section** consists of a much briefer and more practical *'What to do'* section. It summarises the evidence in the form of advice on best practice for the midwife, always including clear criteria for GP referral.

The **third section** comprises a *leaflet* version based on the 'What to do' section but presented in an even briefer format. The full set of leaflets can be easily carried around by midwives working in the community.

HOW TO READ THE GUIDELINES

Section one of each guideline should be read in full at some time, to enable familiarity with the complete evidence base for the management advice given in sections two and three. However, recognising that workload and other circumstances will not always allow the opportunity to read and fully digest this detailed information prior to use, all the sections, as well as each guideline, have been written to 'stand alone'. This facilitates pragmatic use, although those who do read from beginning to end will find some repetition, in particular in describing studies that are applicable to more than one guideline area.

WHEN TO USE THE GUIDELINES

The guidelines were developed for use in the IMPaCT study throughout the whole period of postnatal community midwifery contact, which was up to three months postpartum, although much of the information is likely to be applicable for longer. Some guidelines, however, will be more likely to be used during the first few days (for example Endometritis and abnormal blood loss, Caesarean section wound care), and others at later visits (for example Depression, Backache, Fatigue).

In general the guidelines are for use when a problem is identified, but there are exceptions in relation to the 'initial assessment' sections of three guidelines:

- All women should have an initial assessment in relation to the detection of endometritis and abnormal bleeding (Guideline No. 1).
- All women who had a caesarean section should have an initial assessment of the wound (Guideline No. 3).
- All breastfeeding women should have an initial assessment of feeding to maximise successful breastfeeding (Guideline No. 4).

SYMPTOM IDENTIFICATION CHECKLIST

The guidelines are appropriate when health problems or symptoms are identified, which can be by the midwife observing a problem or the woman (or her partner or family) reporting it. One of the findings of the postpartum morbidity studies, however, was that many health problems had not been reported to the relevant professionals. In order to ensure systematic identification of problems a symptom checklist was used by the midwives in the trial. This was used on about the tenth and twenty eighth postnatal day and at the 10–12 week final consultation, although it would be appropriate for use at other times. A copy of this checklist is included in Appendix 2.

1

Endometritis and abnormal bleeding

INTRODUCTION

Traditionally midwifery postnatal care has included routine assessment of uterine involution and observation of lochia to detect deviations from normal physiological recovery following childbirth. The introduction of antibiotics during the inter-war years, alongside changes in obstetric care, contributed to a reduction in what was previously a high level of maternal mortality and morbidity from puerperal infection and postpartum haemorrhage. Although these conditions remain a major cause of death in developing countries, the priority given in the United Kingdom to routine observations of fundal height has changed and the role of such assessment by midwives questioned (Marchant et al 1996). Health professionals with responsibility for postnatal care are being urged to continue to be vigilant with regard to the development of puerperal infection—14 maternal deaths as a direct consequence of sepsis were recorded during the triennial period 1994–1996 (Department of Health 1998). Even less severe cases can contribute to the high level of morbidity generally experienced by women following childbirth (Glazener et al 1995, MacArthur et al 1991).

The exact nature of the link between abnormal bleeding and uterine infection or endometritis is not clear. Endometritis may be at the root of all cases of abnormal bleeding, but in some cases suspected sepsis is the predominant feature, while in others bleeding may occur in the absence of any evidence of sepsis. Therefore, abnormal bleeding and endometritis are considered separately in this guideline but, given their interrelationship, crossover is inevitable and their management is considered together.

ENDOMETRITIS

Definition

Endometritis (or uterine infection) occurs as a result of contamination of the endometrial cavity with vaginal organisms during labour and delivery. Invasion of the myometrium may occur and the highly vascular environment of the postpartum genital tract predisposes to the development of septicaemia. This can be rapid and overwhelming and 'puerperal fever' was, and in developing countries still is, an important cause of maternal death. Infection can impede the natural process of uterine involution and lead to severe postpartum haemorrhage. Therefore, if infection is not identified and managed early, high rates of morbidity and even mortality can occur.

Studies tend to classify patients as having endometritis only when postpartum fever is found in conjunction with uterine tenderness and foul lochia (Parrott et al 1989, Pirwany & Mahmood 1997). The causal organisms are usually normal inhabitants of the genital tract (Pastorek & Sanders 1991) and gaining a sample for culture without contamination is problematic, so positive culture is not a prerequisite for diagnosis. In practice however, endometritis is effectively the default diagnosis for any febrile illness without other cause in the immediate postpartum period, especially within the first 24 hours.

Pyrexia is defined as an oral temperature elevated above 37.8°C (Miller-Keane 1992). A transient elevation in maternal temperature is not uncommon during the postnatal period, for example among women who experience breast engorgement on or about the third postpartum day (Royal College of Midwives (RCM) 1991), although the aetiology of this is unclear. The genital tract is a primary source of infection at this time, although other sites of infection must be considered (Calhoun & Brost 1995). In the past, midwifery rules and codes of practice regulated care by defining the range of temperature rise which would initiate referral to a medical practitioner. For example, the Central Midwives Board rules of 1962 stated that if a woman had 'a rise of temperature above 99.4°F, on three successive days, or a rise of temperature to 100.4°F, a registered medical practitioner must be summoned'. With subsequent revisions to these rules and codes over the last two decades, there is no longer a defined range for what constitutes pyrexia, but in clinical practice it appears that an increase in temperature to 37.8°C or above on any occasion during the postnatal period requires medical referral. The US Joint Commission on Maternal Welfare provides a standard definition of an increase in maternal temperature to 38°C or above on any two of the first 10 days postpartum, or a temperature of 38.7°C or higher during the first 24 hours as puerperal fever (French & Smaill 2000).

In endometritis, the pyrexia may be associated with generalised malaise or a flu-like illness. Other clinical features include tachycardia, uterine tenderness and offensive vaginal loss.

The threshold for treating as endometritis a pyrexial postpartum woman in whom alternative sources of infection have been excluded, is likely to vary both individually and institutionally. In one study (Parrott et al 1989), irrespective of cause being established, antibiotics were prescribed for all patients with a temperature of 37.8°C for more than 24 hours after a caesarean section.

Frequency of occurrence

Few studies have reported the incidence of postpartum endometritis population. In a retrospective random sample of 2137 patients delivered vaginally at an Iowa hospital over a 14 year period, the rate of endometritis was 1.6% (Ely et al 1996), and a study from Israel of the outcome of 75 947 term and pre-term singleton deliveries between 1980 and 1997 found an endometritis rate of 0.17% following vaginal delivery and 2.63% following caesarean section (Chaim et al 2000). With retrospective reviews, however, it is difficult to be sure that follow-up was complete as women with endometritis may not be readmitted or may be admitted to a different unit.

Lack of a standard definition also makes it difficult to ascertain accurate rates of occurrence and the estimate will be affected by the rigour with which alternative sources of infection are sought in pyrexial postpartum women, and by the level of ascertainment of infection after discharge from hospital.

Alexander et al (1997) suggest that approximately 2% of women are admitted to hospital with complications associated with abnormal vaginal bleeding and/or uterine infection within 12 weeks of delivery. As with other postpartum infections, estimates of occurrence of endometritis are now influenced by the use of prophylactic antibiotics.

Risk factors

The most important risk factor for endometritis is caesarean delivery. Smaill & Hofmeyr (2000) reviewed 66 trials of antibiotic prophylaxis in caesarean section. Endometritis was consistently classified across trials as pyrexia in the absence of another cause. In the control groups, the overall incidence of endometritis in women undergoing elective caesarean section was 6.4%, and 28.6% in women who had an emergency caesarean. The use of antibiotic prophylaxis for both planned and unplanned caesareans had a significant protective effect against endometritis, reducing the rate by two thirds.

Other factors reported to predispose to endometritis after vaginal deliveries, as presented in the background to a protocol for a Cochrane systematic review of treatment regimes, include: bacterial vaginosis; genital cultures positive for anaerobic gram negative bacilli; prolonged rupture of the membranes; the presence of meconium during labour; low infant birth weight and multiple vaginal examinations (French & Smaill 2000). No association between postnatal endometritis and the use of water for pain relief or delivery has been found (Robertson et al 1998).

ABNORMAL BLEEDING

The main terms used to define abnormality in relation to postpartum vaginal loss are abnormal bleeding and secondary postpartum haemorrhage.

Definitions

The definition of normal postnatal vaginal loss has formed the basis for current practice, and any deviation from it would be defined as abnormal bleeding. Textbooks of midwifery and obstetrics suggest that the postpartum vaginal loss (lochia) should no longer be red after the first 7 days and lochia should diminish within 4–8 weeks of delivery (Abbott et al 1997, Howie 1986). However, the evidence base for these assumptions is not described and recent studies suggest that the normal duration and character of vaginal loss postpartum may be much more varied (Marchant et al 1999, Oppenheimer et al 1986, Visness et al 1997).

Oppenheimer et al (1986), in a prospective cohort study, recruited 617 women who delivered a live infant during a 10 week period and interviewed them within 48 hours of delivery. Each was asked to complete a diary sheet for up to 60 days and record one of three categories, lochia rubra (red), serosa (pink) and alba (white), which best described the colour of their lochia. Women were also given a fourth choice to describe when vaginal loss had ceased or normal pre-pregnancy discharge returned. Diary sheets were returned when no loss had been recorded for 7 days, except for recurrence of menses; only 236 women (38%) completed and returned diary sheets. The median duration of lochia rubra was 4 days, and for lochia serosa 22 days; 87 (36%) women did not experience lochia alba, as their loss ceased with lochia serosa. No average duration of lochia alba was given for the remaining 149 women. Results confirmed clinical impressions that lochia persists for longer than is generally anticipated; 15% of women still had lochia serosa at 6 weeks postpartum, and 4% at 60 days. The researchers concluded that prolonged vaginal loss was neither unusual nor abnormal, although some caution should be applied to these findings because of the low response rate.

Visness et al (1997) carried out a prospective study of breastfeeding women in Manila, the Philippines, to examine their experience of postnatal vaginal loss and compare findings with the duration and stages of lochia as described in a commonly used obstetric textbook in the USA. The study was undertaken as part of a randomised controlled trial of the effectiveness of the lactational amenorrhoea method of contraception. All women who chose this method of contraception, had given birth vaginally and had previously breast fed a child for a minimum of 12 months were invited to take part; 477 consented (the total number of eligible women was not given). Follow-up was for 1 year from the day of delivery. The women were given calendars to record daily, starting from the day of delivery, whether they had experienced vaginal bleeding or spotting. The median duration of lochia was 27 days (range 5–90 days) and did not vary by age, parity, infant characteristics or breastfeeding frequency. A quarter of the women reported that blood loss stopped and then recommenced. Lochia lasted for longer than the period of 2 weeks defined in the obstetric textbook and the return of menses was rare before 8 weeks.

It would be difficult to replicate this study in the UK, as few women continue breastfeeding beyond 4 months (Foster et al 1997) and those who do are likely to have socio-demographic characteristics which differ from the general child-bearing population. However, that lochial flow persisted up to and beyond the sixth postnatal week was confirmed by the BLiPP study (Marchant et al 1999). BLiPP was a three part research study to investigate the hypothesis that 'routine abdominal palpation of uterine fundal height in postnatal women from 24 hours after delivery until the midwife discharges the woman from her care, fails to predict abnormal uterine bleeding or uterine infection' (Marchant & Alexander 1996). One aim of the first part of the study was to describe the range of normal vaginal loss from 24 hours until 3 months after delivery.

To collect data for this, a prospective survey of 524 women from two health districts in the South of England was carried out between 1995 and 1996. Women were asked to complete two questionnaires and two diaries at intervals up to 16 weeks post delivery. Information on demographic and delivery characteristics was obtained from birth registers for all eligible women (i.e. women who delivered in the local area and who could speak/read/write English). The first questionnaire was completed between 48 hours and 5 days after delivery, depending on whether study recruitment had taken place on the postnatal ward, or if the woman had been contacted following discharge. Women were asked about their experience of vaginal loss immediately following delivery and about the loss experienced on the day the questionnaire was completed. They were offered a range of descriptions to help them answer questions on the colour and amount of vaginal loss; 350 (67%) women responded. Between days two and ten, 318 (61%) women completed the first diary and 284

(54%) completed the second diary on the fourteenth, twenty first and twenty eighth postnatal days. Women were asked to record details about various aspects of their postnatal health, such as psychological state and infant feeding, as well as the amount and duration of vaginal loss. The second questionnaire, sent 3 months after delivery, included questions on the duration and description of vaginal loss and about any problems associated with prolonged or excessive vaginal loss after the first 28 days up to completion of the questionnaire was completed by 325 (62%) women.

Vaginal loss was more varied in the amount, colour and duration than described in commonly used midwifery textbooks, a similar finding to Visness et al (1997). The duration of vaginal loss ranged from 2 to 86 days after delivery, with a mean of 24 days. Duration was not associated with parity and 6% of women reported vaginal loss from 6 weeks up to 12 weeks postpartum. One interesting finding was that 7 (4%) of the 175 primiparae who returned the first questionnaire were unaware that they would experience blood loss after childbirth. The researchers concluded that findings could be used to inform women and health professionals of the colour, amount and duration of vaginal loss for the first 3 months following childbirth.

Secondary PPH is traditionally defined as a severe blood loss occurring after the first 24 hours of delivery and up to 6 weeks postpartum but there is no precise definition of what constitutes a severe blood loss. That bleeding is 'severe' will sometimes be self-evident, but is mostly subjective at the point where advice is sought. In clinical practice the passage of 'large' blood clots is often used as an indication of potential problems and the term secondary PPH largely used when medical intervention is required. There is no evidence base to show if the size or number of clots passed is indicative of potential or actual morbidity. In the absence of relevant evidence the decision to take further action will continue to be subjective.

Frequency of occurrence

Because the definition of 'severe blood loss' is imprecise, the incidence of significant abnormal bleeding or secondary PPH is difficult to ascertain, as reports may only refer to the most adverse outcomes. Prospective studies were not found and, as with endometritis, retrospective hospital based reviews are likely to be underestimates as patients managed in the community and those admitted to other units will not be included. In one such case note review in Hong Kong, the secondary PPH cases identified formed 0.38% of all deliveries, but the authors gave no details on how complete ascertainment of cases was likely to have been (Fung et al 1996). The rate of secondary PPH cases over a 2 year period between 1978 and 1980 in Detroit was 1.5%, but again no assessment can be made of case ascertainment for this study (Lee et al 1981). Rome estimated the rate of occurrence in his series to be 1.3% (Rome 1975). These estimates are consistent with Alexander et al's (1997) estimate of 2% readmission with abnormal bleeding or uterine infection.

Risk factors

The International Federation of Gynecology and Obstetrics reported the most common causes of secondary PPH to be subinvolution of the placental site, infection and retained products of conception (RPOC) (ACOG 1990). Retained products of conception may provide the focus for infection, or their presence may mechanically inhibit retraction of the uterus. RPOC were found in 17.9% of 106 women with secondary PPH in Rome's (1975) series.

It is likely, however, that excessive bleeding will not always occur with retained products of conception and an ultrasound study supports this (Tekay & Joupila 1993). In some cases of secondary PPH, the primary problem may be failure of the normal process of involution without either infection or RPOC.

Khong & Khong (1993) undertook a case note and histological review of women with postpartum haemorrhage occurring between 24 hours and 6 months following delivery. The purpose of the study was to look for evidence of abnormal placentation in women who had secondary postpartum haemorrhage. In the non-pregnant uterus, the arteries are small in diameter and spiral. In the process of forming the placental bed in pregnancy, these vessels become much larger and more flaccid. Failure of this normal placentation has been linked with fetal growth retardation, pre-eclampsia and other pregnancy conditions (Khong et al 1996, Pijnenborg et al 1991). The authors' aim was to determine evidence of failure of the normal process whereby these vessels collapse and thrombose prior to regeneration of the normal non-pregnant pattern. They called this subinvolution of the placental bed.

The study population was defined by histological material received by the pathology laboratory at one Australian hospital. Therefore, women who were managed conservatively or who had surgery but from whom no material was obtained, were excluded. Of the 169 cases identified over a 5 year period between 1986 and 1991, 109 (64.5%) presented within 6 weeks of delivery and 54 (35.5%) between 6 weeks and 6 months postpartum. Including cases up to 6 months later in the analysis means the findings could relate to a subsequent pregnancy, and the following results relate to the cases presenting within 6 weeks. In 32% (n = 35) of the 109 cases presenting before 6 weeks, retained placental tissue was identified. Evidence of endometritis was adjudged to be present in only 4.6% (n = 5).

The authors classified 20.2% (n = 22) as showing 'subinvolution of placental bed vessels'; the remaining 43.1% (n = 47) specimens were 'non-diagnostic material', normal endometrium, decidua or showed 'normal' placental involution.

The study also attempted to explore associations between this finding and the conditions associated with abnormal placentation during pregnancy. Review of the clinical case notes was undertaken but no associations found.

Uterine involution

In addition to charting postpartum vaginal loss and measuring temperature in an attempt to detect and treat endometritis and secondary postpartum haemorrhage early, much of women's routine postpartum care has been centred on the measurement of uterine involution. Whether failure of involution is a risk factor or an effect of endometritis and postpartum haemorrhage is not clear, but its importance and detection are considered here.

Involution describes the return of the uterus to a pelvic organ and the progress of involution is usually assessed by measurement of the symphysis–fundal distance (S–FD). This is the distance from the top of the uterine fundus to the top of the symphysis pubis. Delayed uterine involution is referred to as subinvolution of the uterus and is diagnosed by perceived delay in the reduction of the size of the uterus. There is limited information about the number of women diagnosed as having subinvolution, the relationship between subinvolution alone and subsequent outcome, the referral rate and the most appropriate management of subinvolution as a solitary sign. Findings from the latter stages of the BLiPP study should give some information on this.

The most commonly used methods to assess involution are anthropometry (simple abdominal palpation) or a tape measure. Midwifery textbooks vary in their description of the rate at which uterine involution occurs and lack detail of how the measurement of fundal height should be obtained (Cluett et al 1995). Nevertheless, failure of the uterus to involute could indicate the presence of retained products of conception. One study, undertaken to describe uterine involution in a small sample of primiparae who had a normal vaginal delivery (n = 28), found considerable variability in the pattern of uterine involution, not only between women but also in the daily rate of decline experienced by individual women (Cluett et al 1997). Twenty two women had at least one episode of 'slow decline' (defined as a decline in the S–FD of <1 cm over 3 or more days) at various times during the puerperium. It is possible that variability in the pattern of decline could be even greater amongst multiparae and those who had a caesarean section.

Because there was no evidence to suggest that midwives could measure S–FD with precision, Cluett et al (1995) investigated intra-observer variability, where the same midwife measured the same women using a tape measure, and inter-observer variability, where different midwives measured the same women. Results showed that there was a significant degree of error in measurement of the S–FD when measurements for the same women were taken repeatedly by the same midwife, and the degree of error was even greater when measurements from the same women were taken by different midwives. The disparity between the inter- and intra-rater observations suggests that measurement of uterine involution is unreliable. The authors concluded that measuring S–FD with a tape measure is not precise enough to enable clinical judgements to be made about normal or abnormal progress of uterine involution, and should be discontinued.

An earlier case control study also assessed the value of the postpartum measurement of the S–FD. Bergstrom & Libombo (1992) compared one group of 51 women who had clinically evident signs of endometritis–myometritis with 51 women matched for age, parity and number of days postpartum who had no signs of infection. They found that there was no significant difference between the S–FD measurements of the two groups. These researchers concluded that an infected uterus does not differ in fundal height from a healthy uterus. However, the findings should be interpreted with caution, as the study did not assess the level of accuracy of measurements obtained and the controls were matched only to within 2 postpartum days.

In making the diagnosis of subinvolution, other factors are usually taken into account such as: the presence of abdominal tenderness; pyrexia; offensive lochia and a change in the nature and amount of lochia.

INVESTIGATION AND MANAGEMENT OF SUSPECTED ENDOMETRITIS OR ABNORMAL BLOOD LOSS

Investigation

Some women with abnormal bleeding or suspected uterine infection will require investigation and will be referred for an ultrasound scan. As a result of the scan findings the woman may undergo evacuation to remove retained products of conception. No controlled trials have been undertaken of the routine use of ultrasound to diagnose accurately the complications of involution or prolonged bleeding (Montgomery & Alexander 1994). Hertzberg & Bowie (1991) reviewed the ultrasound images of 53 postnatal women referred for possible retained products. Ultrasound findings were correlated with clinical and pathological reports on women who underwent an evacuation of retained products of conception (ERPC). Only 11 of 53 women had pathologically proven retained placental tissue. The most common finding in women with confirmed pathology was an echogenic mass in the uterine cavity (n = 9). These authors noted that the interpretation of ultrasound findings should be undertaken by an expert prior to performing curettage.

Studies have shown that, in some cases, debris in the uterine cavity may be normal in the early postnatal period. Tekay & Joupila (1993) carried out a longitudinal study to investigate postnatal alterations in peripheral vascular resistance of uterine arteries. Repeat ultrasound observations were performed on 42 postnatal women who had no symptoms of abnormal bleeding. One finding was the detection of debris in the uterine cavity in 21% of women during the first postpartum week, none of whom experienced subsequent morbidity.

As part of a study which evaluated ultrasound assessment of the uterine cavity postpartum, Carlan et al (1997) scanned 131 women immediately after the placenta was delivered. The 131 women then had their uteri explored manually and with sponge curettage. With a sensitivity for ultrasound of only 44% in detecting RPOC, the authors had to conclude that the appearance of retained products immediately after placental delivery is very variable.

Management

In cases where women are pyrexial, may or may not have excessive blood loss but have other clinical symptoms (pyrexia, offensive lochia, uterine tenderness), antibiotics are usually prescribed and the symptoms managed conservatively. The choice of antibiotic regimen is usually empirical, with a spectrum of coverage which will eradicate the mixture of anaerobic and aerobic organisms potentially involved.

For cases of secondary postpartum haemorrhage where bleeding is obviously severe, resuscitation and admission to hospital is required. If findings suggestive of subinvolution or endometritis are accompanied by moderate or prolonged haemorrhage, surgical intervention to perform uterine curettage continues to be a common method of management.

The need to perform surgery on all women who present with secondary PPH has, however, recently been questioned. Fung et al (1996) conducted a retrospective case note analysis at a hospital in Hong Kong to record the clinical features of 78 women diagnosed over a 3 year period with secondary PPH. No details were given of how long after delivery a diagnosis of secondary PPH was made. 31 women (40%) were treated conservatively with antibiotics and all made a good recovery; 47 (60%) had surgical intervention, but in only 23 cases were retained products found on histology. The authors concluded that half of the women did not require surgery, with caesarean section and a history of pyrexia being the only useful indicators in deciding whether to undertake surgical intervention, suggesting that conservative management should be used. Other observations made were a lack of correlation between the severity and timing of the bleeding and retained products. The authors concluded that further prospective studies are required to test the validity of their findings.

SUMMARY OF THE EVIDENCE USED IN THIS GUIDELINE

- Endometritis should continue to be considered in all women with a postpartum pyrexia, especially if delivery was by caesarean section.
- Recent observational studies have shown more normal variation in the pattern of postpartum vaginal loss than previously described.
- There is no precise definition of what constitutes abnormal bleeding or what amounts to severe blood loss and, therefore, secondary PPH.
- Evidence that routine midwifery assessment of uterine involution and observation of lochia prevent subsequent morbidity is inconclusive, and more information is required. Studies have shown that charting the physical involution of the uterus is subject to intra- and inter-observer error and it appears that as a single sign of potential postpartum haemorrhage or endometritis, delay in uterine involution may be of limited value.
- Ultrasound studies have shown apparent retained products of conception in women who have no signs of morbidity from excessive bleeding or infection. Further studies are required to ascertain the benefit of ultrasound to detect complications of involution or prolonged bleeding.
- One retrospective case note analysis found that conservative management of secondary PPH was appropriate in at least half of the presenting cases. Further prospective studies are required to determine optimal management.
- The results of the second and third stages of the BLiPP study (to identify women who sought medical advice and a case control study) will be published in due course (Marchant, personal communication) and should provide information on some of these issues.

WHAT TO DO

INITIAL ASSESSMENT — ALL WOMEN

- From delivery details note any problems with delivery or completeness of the third stage. Ensure the uterus is well contracted and central. Explain what you are doing and why, encouraging the woman to feel her uterus to increase awareness of body changes during the puerperium. Ask her to describe the pattern of her loss since delivery. Note date and result of last Hb estimate. Personal hygiene should be discussed as appropriate.

- Assess blood loss. Advise that the amount of loss may be heavy during the first few days, but will gradually become less. The duration of lochia may vary. Lochia should have a non-offensive odour.

- Women who report a heavier blood loss after a breast feed should be reassured that this is normal, provided the loss subsides thereafter. Women who report lower abdominal pains suggestive of uterine origin at any time during the postnatal period and who are not breastfeeding should be monitored.

OTHER VISITS

- Ask the woman specifically about her observation of lochia. Other indications (i.e. amount and colour of blood loss, offensive lochia, abdominal tenderness, general malaise, fever) should be taken into account before deciding if uterine palpation is required.

Abnormal bleeding

- Ask the woman when she became concerned about her loss and how frequently pads have required changing (were they soaked or moderately stained? Ask for a quantifiable description of loss, e.g. three inch stain). Ascertain thickness of pads used. Ask her to describe the colour of loss, i.e. was it bright red, dark, medium or light red, or pale pink? Observe loss on the pad the woman is currently wearing. If the woman has passed large clots these should be examined for RPOC. Is the loss offensive now, or has it been offensive?

- Did loss occur following a particular activity, i.e. breastfeeding or on rising from lying down? A heavier blood loss can be associated with some activities—reassure.

- Perform abdominal palpation if loss is unrelated to other activities. If the uterus is central and well contracted, reassure and advise to continue to observe lochia.

- If uterus feels tender, but loss is no longer arrange to visit the following day to assess condition. Advise that if bleeding is excessive in the meantime, the woman must contact the midwife or GP.

- If the uterus is tender and/or the loss is heavy, check temperature, take HVS and refer to GP. A dipstix analysis of urine should also be performed prior to referral, to exclude the possibility of a UTI (refer to guideline 5, Urinary problems).

- If a woman continues to have prolonged heavy blood loss (more than a heavy period), but no evidence of infection or subinvolution, she should be asked at subsequent visits about her general wellbeing. It may be helpful to check her last Hb result. A woman who is symptomatic of anaemia should be referred to her GP.

Offensive lochia

- Confirm lochia are offensive. Is the colour of the lochia different from previously? Have any blood clots been passed? Exclude infected perineal wound, or poor personal hygiene.

- Check the woman's temperature, ask about systemic symptoms of infection (flu-like symptoms) and gently palpate her abdomen. If she is pyrexial and/or has severe abdominal or pelvic pain, take HVS and dipstix analysis of urine and refer to GP. This action should be taken even if other observations are within expected normal range, but her lochia are offensive.

Pyrexia (temperature >37.8°C)

- If a woman is unwell or complains of flu-like symptoms, take her temperature. If pyrexial, exclude other symptoms which may present with a pyrexia (breast problems, possible UTI, perineal/abdominal wound infection, etc.).

- If the pyrexia is not associated with other symptoms, gently palpate the abdomen; is there uterine pain during palpation? Are lochia heavy and/or offensive, have any large blood clots been passed? If infection is suspected take HVS and dipstix analysis of urine and refer immediately to GP.

- Even if there are no findings to indicate the presence of infection, the decision to refer to the GP must remain at the midwife's discretion.

Abdominal tenderness

- Obtain history of onset and ask about condition of lochia. Gently palpate abdomen to establish the site of pain and assess involution. Is there any lower abdominal pain or generalised tenderness? Is the uterus positioned centrally or deviated, bulky or well contracted (findings could relate to number of postpartum days)? If subinvolution is suspected, take HVS and dipstix analysis of urine. Refer immediately to GP.

Subinvolution

- If you do decide to plot the course of involution and suspect delay, explore the other symptoms and signs of infection or haemorrhage and take action as appropriate.

Severe, life-threatening haemorrhage

If a woman is experiencing a severe haemorrhage at home the aim of immediate care must be to achieve prompt arrest of bleeding before the situation is critical.

- Medical aid must be summoned immediately (ambulance with paramedic support).

- Massaging the uterus will aid expulsion of any clots and cause it to contract.

- If there is time, empty the bladder with an indwelling catheter. Administer ergometrine 0.5 mg IM or IV if trained to do so (unless contraindicated, for example if woman has cardiovascular condition). If trained to do so, commence IV infusion.

- The obstetric unit should be informed of the admission.
- Information and reassurance should be given to the woman and her partner.
- Record all action taken.

GENERAL ADVICE

- It is advisable to wear maternity size pads initially. These should be changed frequently. Based on common practice, pads should be changed each time the toilet is visited or at least four times a day.
- The amount of blood loss (lochia) may be very heavy during the first few days, but it will gradually become less. The duration of lochia may vary. Lochia should have a non-offensive smell.
- The midwife should be contacted if there is a recurrence of bright red fresh loss after the first postpartum week; if a large blood clot is passed on more than one occasion; if loss becomes heavier or offensive.

SUMMARY GUIDELINE

ENDOMETRITIS AND ABNORMAL BLEEDING

INITIAL ASSESSMENT—ALL WOMEN

- Ensure uterus is well contracted and central
- Assess blood loss
- Note problems with delivery or third stage completeness

SUMMON MEDICAL AND PARAMEDICAL SUPPORT IF:

- Severe, life threatening haemorrhage

IMMEDIATE REFERRAL TO THE GP IS REQUIRED IF:

- Suspected uterine infection
- Offensive lochia

SEVERE LIFE THREATENING HAEMORRHAGE

- Summon medical aid immediately via emergency services
- Massage uterus
- Insert indwelling urinary catheter
- IV access
- Administer ergometrine if appropriate

If a deviation from normal uterine recovery is suspected, a detailed history should enable a preliminary diagnosis to be made and appropriate action to be taken. The mother's baseline observations should be checked. A mother with pyrexia (temperature >37.8°C) or abdominal tenderness may be experiencing these subsequent to one of the diagnoses presented below.

Table 1.1 Summary of midwifery care for endometritis and abnormal bleeding

Midwifery care	Abnormal bleeding	Offensive lochia
Establish	• Length of time heavier loss experienced	• Lochia are offensive
Exclude	• Associations with other factors, e.g. breastfeeding, rising up from lying or sitting	• Associations with other factors, e.g. infected perineal wound • Poor personal hygiene
Ask the woman	• To describe amount of loss in inches or centimetres of spread on pad • Is colour of loss different from previously? • Is the loss offensive now, or has it been?	• Is colour of loss different from previously?
Describe and record	• Look at current pad • Identify absorption level of pad used • Describe the size of any clots passed, examine for placental tissues or membranes	

Record temperature and palpate uterus

ACTION	If normal:	If abnormal—raised temperature and/or pulse or uterine tenderness:
	• Reassure • Monitor	• HVS • MSU • Refer to GP • Advise mother about action taken and to contact midwife if symptoms become more severe

GENERAL ADVICE

- Change maternity pads regularly
- Blood loss may be heavy for the first few days, but it will gradually become less. It should have a non-offensive smell
- The midwife should be contacted if the loss becomes:
— heavier
— bright red *after* the first week of delivery
— if a large clot passed on more than one occasion
— offensive

REFERENCES

Abbott H, Bick D, MacArthur C 1997 Health after birth. In: Henderson C, Jones K (eds) Essential midwifery. Mosby, London

Alexander J, Garcia J, Marchant S 1997 The BLiPP study. A joint collaboration between the University of Portsmouth and the National Perinatal Epidemiology Unit, Oxford. Final Report to South & West NHS Executive Research and Development Committee, Feb. Unpublished. Available from the authors.

American College of Obstetricians and Gynecologists (ACOG) Technical Bulletin 1990 Diagnosis and management of postpartum haemorrhage. Int J Gynecol Obstet 36: 159–163

Bergstrom S, Libombo A 1992 Puerperal measurement of the symphysis–fundus distance. Gynecol Obstet Invest 34(2): 76–78

Calhoun B C, Brost B 1995 Emergency management of sudden puerperal fever. Obstet Gynecol Clin N Am 22(2): 357–367

Carlan S J, Scott W T, Pollack R, Harris K 1997 Appearance of the uterus by ultrasound immediately after placental delivery with pathologic correlation. J Clin Ultrasound 25(6): 301–308

Central Midwives Board 1962 Handbook incorporating the rules of the Central Midwives Board, 25th edn. William Clowes, London, p 60

Chaim W, Basiri A, Bar-David J et al 2000 Prevalence and clinical significance of postpartum endometritis and wound infection. Infect Dis Obstet Gynecol 8(2): 72–82

Cluett E R, Alexander J, Pickering R M 1995 Is measuring the symphysis–fundal distance worthwhile? Midwifery 11(4): 174–183

Cluett E R, Alexander J, Pickering R M 1997 What is the normal pattern of uterine involution? An investigation of postpartum uterine involution measured by the distance between the symphysis pubis and the uterine fundus using a tape measure. Midwifery 13: 9–16

Department of Health 1998 Why mothers die. Report on confidential enquiries into maternal deaths in the United Kingdom 1994–1996. The Stationery Office, London

Ely J W, Dawson J D, Townsend A S et al 1996 Benign fever following vaginal delivery. J Fam Pract 43(2): 146–151

Foster K, Lader D, Cheesbrough S 1997 Infant feeding 1995. The Stationery Office. London

French L M, Smaill F M 2000 Antibiotic regimens for endometritis after delivery. Cochrane Review 3. The Cochrane Library, Oxford

Fung E S M, Sin S Y, Tang L 1996 Secondary postpartum haemorrhage: curettage or not? J Obstet Gynaecol 16(6): 514–517

Glazener C M A, Abdalla M, Stroud P et al 1995 Postnatal maternal morbidity: extent, causes, prevention and treatment. Br J Obstet Gynaecol 102(4): 282–287

Hertzberg B, Bowie J 1991 Ultrasound of the postpartum uterus. J Ultrasound Med 10: 451–456

Howie P W 1986 The puerperium and its complications. In: Whitfield C R (ed) Dewhirst's textbook of obstetrics and gynaecology for postgraduates. Blackwell Scientific Publications, Oxford

Khong T Y, Khong T K 1993 Delayed postpartum haemorrhage: a morphologic study of causes and their relation to other pregnancy disorders. Obstet Gynecol 82(1): 17–22

Khong T Y, De Wolf F, Robertsone W B et al 1986 Inadequate vascular response to placentation in pregnancies complicated by pre-eclampsia and by small-for-gestational age infants. Br J Obstet Gynaecol 93: 1049–1059

Lee C Y, Madrazo B, Drukker B H 1981 Ultrasonic evaluation of the postpartum uterus in the management of postpartum bleeding. Obstet Gynecol 58(2): 227–232

MacArthur C, Lewis M, Knox E G 1991 Health after childbirth. HMSO, London

Marchant S, Alexander J 1996 Midwives' assessment of postnatal uterine involution—is it of value? International Congress of Midwives, Conference Proceedings, 24th Triennial Conference Oslo, p 402

Marchant S, Alexander J, Garcia J 1996 Postnatal observations (letter). Midwives 109(1302): 204

Marchant S, Alexander J, Garcia J et al 1999 A survey of women's experiences of vaginal loss from 24 hours to 3 months after childbirth (the BLiPP study). Midwifery 15: 72–81

Miller-Keane 1992 Encyclopaedia and Dictionary of Medicine, Nursing and Allied Health, 5th edn. W B Saunders, Philadelphia

Montgomery E, Alexander J 1994 Assessing postnatal uterine involution: a review and a challenge. Midwifery 10: 73–76

Oppenheimer L W, Sherriff E A, Goodman J D S et al 1986 The duration of lochia. Br J Obstet Gynaecol 93: 754–757

Parrott T, Evans A J, Lowes A et al 1989 Infection following caesarean section. J Hosp Infect 13: 349–354

Pastorek J G, Sanders C V 1991 Antibiotic therapy for postcaesarean endomyometritis. Rev Infect Dis 13(suppl 9): S752–S757

Pijnenborg R, Anthony J, Davey D A et al 1991 Placental bed spiral arteries in the hypertensive disorders of pregnancy. Br J Obstet Gynaecol 98: 648–655

Pirwany I R, Mahmood T 1997 Audit of infective morbidity following caesarean section at a district general hospital. J Obstet Gyaencol 17(5): 439–443

Robertson P A, Huang L J, Croughan-Minihane M S et al 1998 Is there an association between water baths during labor and the development of chorioamnionitis or endometritis? Am J Obstet Gynecol 178(6): 1215–1221

Rome R M 1975 Secondary postpartum haemorrhage. J Obstet Gynaecol 82: 289–292

Royal College of Midwives 1991 Successful breastfeeding, 2nd edn. Churchill Livingstone, Edinburgh

Smaill F, Hofmeyr G J 2000 Antibiotic prophylaxis for Caesarean section. Cochrane Review 3. The Cochrane Library, Oxford

Tekay A, Joupila P 1993 A longitudinal doppler ultrasonographic assessment of the alterations in peripheral vascular resistance of the uterine arteries and ultrasonographic findings of the involuting uterus during the puerperium. Am J Obs Gynecol 168: 190–198

Visness C M, Kennedy K I, Ramos R 1997 The duration and character of postpartum bleeding among breast-feeding women. Obstet Gynecol 89(2): 159–163

Perineal pain and dyspareunia

INTRODUCTION

The majority of women who have a vaginal delivery will experience some degree of perineal pain, which is one of the most commonly reported symptoms in the immediate postnatal period (Sleep 1995). Dyspareunia or painful sexual intercourse, although a different symptom, may be related to perineal pain. Several of the relevant studies, especially those with information on risk factors, have investigated both of these symptoms. If each symptom were to be reviewed and described separately in this guideline, there would be substantial repetition. Some parts of the guideline, therefore, describe perineal pain and dyspareunia in separate sections and others describe them together. Recent data on other sexual health problems after childbirth and on the timing of the resumption of sexual intercourse, is also described/referred to where relevant.

Definitions

Perineal pain is defined as any pain occurring in the perineal body, an area of muscular and fibrous tissue which extends from the symphysis pubis to the coccyx (Kettle 1999). *Dyspareunia* refers to pain or discomfort occurring during sexual intercourse, including pain on penetration. Dyspareunia is sometimes categorised as superficial or deep.

Frequency of occurrence: perineal pain

Information on the prevalence of perineal pain is available from a few observational studies based on representative samples and with adequate response rates. Several trials investigating various forms of perineal management that include perineal pain as an outcome measure have also provided some data, although it is important to keep in mind that whilst trials provide best evidence on causality, where trial inclusion is restricted to particular types of delivery, this limits the generalisability of the prevalence estimates.

In a prospective observational study in Scotland, among a representative sample of all deliveries over a defined period, 42% of 1249 women reported a painful perineum when questioned in hospital (Glazener et al 1995). In the West Berkshire Perineal Management Trial (see p. 23 below), 23% of almost 900 women (inclusion restricted to those expected to have a spontaneous vaginal delivery (SVD)) reported perineal pain at 10 days postpartum (Sleep et al 1984). Among over 5000 spontaneous vaginal births in the 'hands on or poised' trial (HOOP), which compared alternative methods of conducting the second stage of labour, 33% of women in the trial as a whole reported perineal pain in the previous 24 hours, when asked at 10 days postpartum (McCandlish et al 1998).

Perineal pain is clearly very common in the early puerperium, but for some women it can also be more persistent, and various studies have shown that at least 8–10% of women experience this well past the 6 week postnatal discharge from maternity care. In the trial by Sleep et al (1984), when followed up at 3 months, 8% of the women reported perineal pain at that time. In the study by Glazener et al (1995), when questioned again at 8 weeks, 22% of the sample reported experiencing a painful perineum between then and the first week; and when questioned at 12–18 months, 9.8% had experienced perineal pain some time between 8 weeks and 12–18 months. Brown & Lumley (1998) contacted 1336 women at 6–7 months postpartum in a cross-sectional study of all deliveries occurring over 2 weeks within a region in Australia, and found that for 21% a painful perineum had been a problem at some time since the birth. The proportion who still had this at 6–7 months was not given.

Frequency of occurrence: dyspareunia

As with perineal pain, there is information on the prevalence of dyspareunia from observational studies and from the trials of perineal management, although again it must be remembered that data on this from samples restricted to particular delivery types or parity groups.

Brown & Lumley (1998), in the Australian study described earlier, found that 26% of the women questioned at 6–7 months postpartum had experienced 'a sexual problem' some time since the birth, although further specification of the problem was not given nor what proportion still had it. Glazener (1997) found that at 8 weeks postpartum 25% of the sample had not attempted intercourse. The remaining 75% had attempted intercourse, although for 5% it had been unsuccessful. Questions on problems with intercourse were included, showing that between 1 and 8 weeks 28% of women had found intercourse to be sore or difficult; between 2 and 18 months this was reported by 20%. Lack of interest in sex was reported by 9% of women at 8 weeks, rising to 21% between 2 and 18 months.

A recent cross-sectional study of all primiparous women delivering in one maternity unit in London was conducted to enquire about a range of sexual health problems (Barrett et al 2000). Postal questionnaires were sent at 6 months postpartum to 796 primiparae asking about sexual problems since the birth and prior to pregnancy; 484 (61%) replied. By 6 weeks (as recalled) 32% of women had resumed intercourse, 62% had done so by 8 weeks and 81% by 3 months. Dyspareunia, which was specified as including painful penetration and/or pain during intercourse or orgasm, was experienced by 62% of women at some time in the first 3 months after birth and 31% still had this at 6 months. Loss of sexual desire was reported by 53% of women in the first 3 months, and by 37% at 6 months. Other problems still experienced at 6 months were vaginal tightness (20%), vaginal looseness or lack of muscle tone (12%) and lack of vaginal lubrication (26%). In relation to the year before pregnancy and, although subject to greater recall bias, all sexual problems were found to have increased significantly in the first 3 months after delivery. Although all problems had declined by 6 months postpartum, they were still substantially greater than pre-pregnancy levels. The response rate in this survey was 61%, which is good given the sensitive nature of the subject, but gives less confidence in relation to prevalence estimates. Even if all of the non-responders were problem-free, however, the findings still provide clear evidence that sexual problems are common as well as persistent following childbirth.

Sleep et al (1984), in their trial, found that by 3 months postpartum 90% of women reported having resumed sexual intercourse. Just over half of these had experienced dyspareunia at some time since the birth and almost 20% still had it at 3 months. Klein et al (1994), in a similar trial (see p. 24 below), found that 64% of the sample had resumed intercourse by 6 weeks and 96% by 3 months. On first intercourse almost 80% of the women reported some pain, although in most cases this was only mild or discomforting.

Risk factors: perineal pain and dyspareunia

The main risk factors of perineal pain and dyspareunia identified in studies relate to mode of delivery, perineal trauma and primiparity. Since these factors are all highly interrelated, appropriate multivariate analyses need to be undertaken in order to report on the independent effects of each. Methods of managing perineal trauma, such as the use of different suture methods and materials, have also been investigated with respect to subsequent perineal pain and dyspareunia and are described in this section on risk factors.

Mode of delivery

Mode of delivery is associated with substantial variation in perineal pain (short and long term), with much higher rates occurring after instrumental compared with spontaneous vaginal deliveries and the lowest rates occurring after caesarean sections. Similar differences for dyspareunia also occur but are generally less marked.

In the study by Glazener et al (1995) described earlier, differences in perineal pain according to delivery mode were clearly documented, occurring whilst still in hospital, between then and 8 weeks, and between 2 and 18 months. The respective prevalences whilst in hospital were 84% after instrumental delivery, 42% after an SVD, and 5% after caesarean section; 59%, 19% and 4% between then and 8 weeks; and 30%, 7% and 2% between 2 and 18 months. Data on dyspareunia were also reported for this sample (see p. 20), but not separately according to mode of delivery (Glazener 1997).

Johanson et al (1993) obtained data on a number of morbidity indicators from 313 women who were part of a randomised controlled trial (RCT) of forceps versus vacuum extraction deliveries, and from 100 consecutive unselected SVDs. A significant difference in perineal discomfort at 24–48 hours was found, which occurred in 45% of the instrumental delivery group and 28% of the SVD group (odds ratio (OR) 2.1, 95% confidence interval (CI) 1.2–3.4). At 15–24 months postpartum, 28% compared with 19% respectively reported a painful perineum (mostly occurring only sometimes), but this difference was not statistically significant. Pain on intercourse (mostly occurring only sometimes) at 15–24 months, however, was significantly more common in the instrumental group, reported by 37% compared with 21% of the spontaneous vaginal deliveries (OR 2.0, 95% CI 1.03–3.80).

Brown & Lumley (1998), in their population-based sample in Australia, found that perineal pain, reported as a problem some time between the birth and 6–7 months postpartum, occurred in 20% of women after SVD, 54% after instrumental birth, 2% after emergency caesarean section and none after elective section (OR for instrumental relative to SVD 4.69, 95% CI 3.2–6.8). Sexual problems (not further specified) differed only for instrumental deliveries, being reported by 24%, 39%, 29% and 27% respectively after the four types of delivery (OR for instrumental relative to SVD 2.06, 95% CI 1.4–3.0). These differences in perineal pain and sexual problems between instrumental compared with spontaneous vaginal births were adjusted to take account of infant birthweight, length of labour and degree of perineal trauma, and remained statistically significant.

Barrett et al (2000), in their study of sexual problems among primiparae, found that dyspareunia occurring some time during the first 3 months was reported by 62% of women after SVD, 78% after forceps/ventouse delivery,

41% after a section with labour and 47% after a section without labour. After logistic regression, the difference for forceps/ventouse deliveries relative to SVD remained significant (OR 2.41, 95% CI 1.24–4.69), but the differences for both types of caesarean section did not. Dyspareunia at 6 months postpartum was reported by 30% of women after SVD, 37% after forceps/ventouse, and 28% and 21% respectively after section with and without labour, but none of these differences was statistically significant. Continued breastfeeding up to 6 months was one of the two factors in this study found to be significantly associated with dyspareunia at 6 months. The other was a previous history of dyspareunia prior to pregnancy and both factors remained significant after logistic regression. Among the women still breastfeeding, 40% reported dyspareunia compared with 25% of those not breastfeeding (OR 2.25, 95% CI 1.42–3.57). The researchers suggest that hormone levels, loss of libido and vaginal dryness could contribute towards the symptom excess in breastfeeding mothers.

Glazener (1997) found that women who were still breastfeeding at 8 weeks were significantly more likely to report a lack of interest in intercourse than those who were bottle feeding. Tiredness was also more common among the breastfeeding mothers, but even after taking account of this, the relationship with lack of interest in sex remained.

Perineal trauma

Perineal trauma is generally considered to be more likely to result in perineal pain and dyspareunia than if the perineum is intact, but there has been considerable debate on the benefits and adverse effects of episiotomy compared with spontaneous laceration (Sleep 1995). Several trials have examined this issue. The West Berkshire Perineal Management Trial (Sleep et al 1984), referred to earlier, of a restricted versus a liberal episiotomy policy, was the first to provide good evidence on the effects of episiotomy use among women who, towards the end of second stage labour, were expected to have a spontaneous vaginal delivery. For women allocated to the restrictive group, the midwife was asked to avoid episiotomy and only perform an incision if fetal indications (bradycardia, tachycardia, meconium stained liquor) warranted this (n = 498). In the liberal group the midwife was asked to try to prevent a perineal tear (n = 502), the intention being that she should use episiotomy more liberally to do this. The different policies did result in more tears and more intact perinea in the restrictive group, but no differences were found in perineal pain at 10 days or 3 months, nor in dyspareunia at 3 months. These authors concluded that the findings provide little support for either the liberal use of episiotomy or for claims that its reduced use would decrease postpartum morbidity (Sleep et al 1984).

Klein et al (1994) carried out a similar trial in Canada, which again found that although significantly fewer episiotomies were performed in the restrictive policy group, there were no differences at 1 and 10 days postpartum in perineal pain, or in sexual problems (pain and sexual satisfaction) at 3 months.

Since these trials a Cochrane systematic review has been undertaken (Carroli et al 2000), including four other randomised controlled trials comparing policies of the restrictive use of episiotomy versus routine/liberal use, confirmed that there were no differences in perineal pain or dyspareunia according to episiotomy policy, although other differences (reduced risk of posterior perineal trauma, less suturing and fewer healing complications) led the reviewers to conclude that a restrictive episiotomy policy was beneficial and should be recommended.

Since these trials were comparing perineal management policies, some women in the restricted episiotomy group still had an episiotomy, and vice versa. In the study by Klein et al (1994), it was felt that this justified undertaking further subgroup analyses and all women in the trial were recategorised (irrespective of trial group allocation) according to the type of perineal trauma (intact, laceration, episiotomy, third and fourth degree tears). Perineal pain between days 1 and 10 and at 3 months was found to be least in the intact group and greatest in those with third and fourth degree tears. Episiotomy and spontaneous tears were intermediate and differed from each other for early perineal pain and for later pain classed as occurring most or all of the time, both a little more common after episiotomy. Dyspareunia on first resumption of intercourse followed a similar pattern of relationship with trauma. The type of episiotomy in this trial was midline, which is rarely practised in the UK, and almost all women in the trial had spontaneous vaginal deliveries.

In a subsequent analysis of data from the study by Glazener (1997) to determine the independent predictors of pain or difficulty with intercourse at 2 months postpartum, logistic regression showed episiotomy to be an independent predictor of this (Glazener 1998).

Parity

Perineal pain and dyspareunia have both been documented as more common after first compared with subsequent births (Barrett et al 1998, Glazener et al 1995). However, the extent to which this is influenced by the greater proportion of instrumental deliveries and perineal trauma that occur among first births is difficult to assess. The parity association found by Glazener et al (1995) for painful perineum was based on univariate analysis, not taking other factors into account. For pain or difficulty with intercourse at 2 months postpartum, multivariate analysis, to take account of possible interrelated factors, showed that primiparity remained associated with the symptoms, although forceps delivery did not. In the perineal management trial by Sleep et al (1984), data were presented separately for first and later births showing mild and moderate perineal pain at 10 days reported by almost twice as many primiparae as multiparae. This study was of anticipated spontaneous vaginal births so should not be confounded by any parity-related instrumental delivery effect, but in both trial arms the primiparae had more perineal trauma (episiotomy or laceration) than the multiparae. Klein et al (1994), in their similar study, stated that primiparae experienced more perineal pain and sexual problems than multiparae, but presented no data on this.

Suture materials and methods

The effects of suture materials and methods on subsequent perineal pain and dyspareunia have been examined in a number of randomised controlled trials, some of which have had clear findings relevant to practice.

A Cochrane systematic review, including eight randomised controlled trials, compared synthetic suture materials with catgut (Kettle & Johanson 2000a). Catgut is manufactured from collagen from mammals, and has been a commonly used suture material, whilst the synthetic suture materials polyglycolic acid (Dexon) and polyglactin (Vicryl) are more recent. All the trials in the Cochrane review were consistent in showing lower rates of short term (3 days) perineal pain in the synthetic suture groups (OR 0.62, 95% CI 0.54–0.71). Two of the trials examined perineal pain and three examined dyspareunia at 3 months, with no differences found in either of these longer term outcomes according to type of suture material. Other outcomes, i.e. the need for analgesia, and suture dehiscence, were reduced in the groups sutured with synthetic material, but two trials that included as secondary outcomes the removal of suture material at 10 days and 3 months found this was undertaken more often in the synthetic materials group. The reviewers concluded that the use of absorbable synthetic suture material (polyglycolic acid and polyglactin sutures) appears to decrease short term perineal pain. The length of time taken for synthetic material to be absorbed, however, is of concern (Kettle & Johanson 2000a).

The effects of continuous subcuticular versus interrupted transcutaneous sutures for closure of perineal skin on long and short term pain and dyspareunia (as well as other outcomes) was examined in another Cochrane systematic review which included four trials (Kettle & Johanson 2000b). Three trials examined short term pain (Banninger et al 1978, Isager-Sally et al 1986, Mahomed et al 1989), all of which found lower rates in the continuous suturing groups, the meta-analysis of these showing statistical significance (OR 0.68, 95% CI 0.53–0.86). Only one trial examined long term pain (Mahomed et al 1989), and found no difference according to suture method.

Dyspareunia at 3 months was examined in three of the trials, the meta-analysis of which showed no significant difference according to suture methods. Two of these trials had found *lower* rates of dyspareunia in the continuous suture group, although in only one (very small trial) was this significant: the third showed significantly *higher* rates, which might have been explained by the fact that a greater proportion of the women in the continuous suture group in this trial had resumed intercourse by 3 months. Failure to resume pain-free intercourse by 3 months postpartum was examined in one trial, showing no difference according to suture method. Other outcomes, i.e. the need for analgesia or resuturing, did not differ between suture methods but there was less need for the removal of sutures in the continuous technique group. The conclusion of the reviewers was that the subcuticular perineal repair technique may be associated with less perineal pain in the immediate postpartum period than the interrupted technique, but long term effects are less clear (Kettle & Johanson 2000b).

A recent stratified randomised controlled trial (Ipswich Childbirth Study—included in the systematic review of type of suture material described above) used a 2×2 factorial design and also compared the effects of the standard three stage suturing method with a two stage method, in which the perineal skin was left unsutured (Gordon et al 1998). The trial was carried out in a single centre and involved 1780 women of all parities who sustained episiotomy or first or second degree tears following spontaneous or instrumental vaginal deliveries. Women were assessed by questionnaire at 24–48 hours, 10 days and at 3 months postpartum. No differences were found in perineal pain at 24–48 hours or 10 days between the two and three stage repair groups, but at 3 months fewer women in the two stage group reported perineal pain and more had resumed pain-free intercourse. Among women who had resumed intercourse, reduced rates of dyspareunia in the two stage group just reached statistical significance (relative risk (RR) 0.80, 95% CI 0.65–0.99).

Another variation in perineal management during spontaneous vaginal delivery has been evaluated in a recent RCT, which included perineal pain at 10 days as the main outcome measure and pain and dyspareunia at 3 months as additional outcomes (McCandlish et al 1998). This was the HOOP trial ('hands on or poised'), in which 5471 women were randomised to being delivered with the 'hands on' (the midwife put pressure on the baby's head and 'guarded' the perineum; n = 2731) or the 'hands poised' method (the midwife kept her hands poised, not touching the baby's head or the perineum, allowing spontaneous delivery of the shoulders; n = 2740). At 10 days postpartum significantly more women in the 'hands poised' group (34.1%) reported perineal pain in the previous 24 hours compared with the 'hands on' group (31.1%), although this difference was greatest in the 'mild' pain category. There was no difference, however, in perineal pain or in dyspareunia at 3 months. Other outcomes, including urinary problems, bowel problems and postnatal depression, did not vary between groups, but episiotomy rates were significantly higher in the 'hands on' group, and manual removal of the placenta was significantly lower.

Management: perineal pain

Local applications for pain relief

A survey of 50 maternity units by Sleep & Grant (1988a) found that the majority reported ice packs to be the most frequently used local application for the relief of perineal pain, used in 84% of units; 'Epifoam' (Stafford-Miller Ltd) was used in over half of the units and ultrasound therapy in over a third. Moore & James (1989) conducted a randomised controlled trial of three topical pain relief applications (witchhazel, ice and Epifoam) in 300 women who had episiotomy for a forceps delivery. The women were randomly assigned to one of the three groups at delivery and the first application of the agent was made immediately following perineal repair. Women were advised they could use the agent at any time following this. 34 women were excluded from follow-up because the trial protocol was not adhered to, and complete data were only available for 205 women who had inpatient assessment of pain. A hospital appointment for the 6 week postnatal check was attended by 126 women, at which information was obtained on resumption of intercourse and the perineal wound examined. There were no differences in pain relief achieved amongst the three groups on the first day post delivery, and at 6 weeks among those who attended the hospital there were no differences in the timing of resumption of first intercourse, wound healing and resolution of perineal pain.

A survey of perineal care carried out by the National Childbirth Trust (NCT) (Greenshields & Hulme 1993) also found that ice packs were the most commonly offered local application for pain relief. Whilst ice packs appear to give immediate symptomatic relief, there is no evidence of long term benefits and it is suggested that, in theory, vasoconstriction may actually delay wound healing (Sleep 1995). 'Ice burns' may also be sustained if packs are applied in direct contact with the skin. A pad containing cooling gel which can be moulded around the perineum has recently been developed, but evidence of the effectiveness of this is required and studies are ongoing (Steen & Cooper 1998).

The effects of administering a local anaesthetic versus a placebo to relieve perineal pain were assessed in one small trial of 103 primiparous women (Harrison & Brennan 1987). Results showed that 5% lidocaine (lignocaine) spray and gel was associated with more effective pain relief than the placebo at 10 days after delivery, but health care staff were not blinded to group allocation, which could have resulted in observer bias.

Oral analgesia

In the survey by Sleep & Grant (1988a) (described above), oral analgesia (usually paracetamol) was the first line treatment for mild perineal pain in 78% of the 50 maternity units investigated. Sleep (1995), in a review of postnatal perineal care, noted that several factors need to be considered when deciding on the most appropriate oral preparation, including: an assessment of the severity of the pain; the potential for the analgesia to be secreted into breast milk; and possible side effects, such as constipation or nausea.

Among the women in the NCT survey (Greenshields & Hulme 1993) who had used oral analgesia to relieve perineal pain, the majority considered paracetamol to be the most effective. Other oral analgesia taken by women in this survey included aspirin, ibuprofen, codeine and co-proxamol. Effectiveness of simple oral analgesia is considered in more detail in guideline 3 under pain relief following caesarean section.

Diclofenac suppositories

There have been two trials showing that diclofenac suppositories, used prophylactically after perineal trauma, can be effective in the short term relief of perineal pain. One trial randomly allocated 110 women who had episiotomy during spontaneous vaginal delivery to receive a diclofenac suppository (n = 56) or a placebo (n = 54), immediately following episiotomy repair (Yoong et al 1997). The women completed a visual analogue score (VAS) and a modified pain score to assess pain at 24 and 48 hours, and a review of prescription charts was undertaken to assess the need for additional analgesia. At 24 hours the women randomised to receive diclofenac had less pain, although at 48 hours there were no pain score differences between the groups. Those who received diclofenac, however, required less additional analgesia throughout the 48 hour period.

Similar results were found in the other randomised controlled trial, which included repair of either episiotomy or second degree tear (Searles & Pring 1998). Diclofenac suppository or placebo was given at the time of perineal repair and 12 hours later. 100 women were randomised but results were based on 89 women who completed follow-up. Pain scores were assessed at 12, 24, 48 and 72 hours after delivery, using a scale where 0 = no pain and 5 = worst pain possible. In the diclofenac group, the mean pain score was less than in the control group at each time interval, and the women were less likely to have required additional analgesia, an effect which also persisted to final pain scores assessment at 72 hours.

Although both these trials were small, results suggest that prophylactic rectal diclofenac following second degree tear or episiotomy for spontaneous vaginal delivery is beneficial and the effect appears to persist into the second and third postpartum days. Larger studies are required to confirm this, and to assess benefits in women with perineal trauma following instrumental delivery and whether this route confers any advantage over oral administration (Oxford Pain Internet Site 2001).

Bathing

One small trial compared the effects on perineal pain of sitting in either warm or cold baths (Ramler & Roberts 1986). This found that whilst cold baths were significantly more effective in relieving perineal pain, especially straight after delivery, the effect was limited to the first half hour of treatment and few women would want to sit in a cold bath—119 of 159 women approached refused to take part in the trial.

A remedy traditionally considered to relieve perineal pain and enhance wound healing has been the addition of salt to bath water. A three arm randomised controlled trial examined the effectiveness of adding salt, a 25 ml sachet of Savlon or nothing to the bath water each day for the first 10 days, among 1800 vaginal deliveries (Sleep & Grant 1988b). The prevalence of perineal pain and pattern of wound healing at 10 days were similar in all groups and at 3 months perineal pain still did not differ, nor did timing of resumption of intercourse or dyspareunia. Using salt or Savlon bath additives, therefore, cannot be recommended to reduce pain or dyspareunia or to enhance healing, but over 90% of women in each of the groups reported at 10 days that they had found bathing to be helpful in relieving their perineal discomfort.

Alternative therapies

There is anecdotal evidence from women that some alternative remedies, such as arnica and lavender oil, provide relief of perineal pain (Greenshields & Hulme 1993). Dale & Cornwell (1994) conducted a randomised controlled trial involving 635 women, which compared pure lavender oil, synthetic lavender oil or an inert oil added to bath water on each of the first 10 days postpartum. Daily discomfort scores were assessed using a visual analogue scale but no significant differences between the groups were found. Further trials are required to assess the safety and benefit of alternative remedies before they can be recommended as effective for the relief of perineal pain.

Ultrasound

There is some evidence of the effectiveness of ultrasound in the treatment of soft tissue injuries from general population studies (Binder et al 1985), and ultrasound and pulsed electromagnetic therapy are now increasingly used as treatments to relieve acute perineal pain. Ultrasound is thought to reduce pain by resolution of the inflammation process and reduction of pressure from haematoma and oedema on pain sensitive structures (Hay-Smith 2000). In the survey of obstetric units described earlier (Sleep & Grant 1988a), 36% reported using ultrasound and 6% pulsed electromagnetic therapy.

Hay-Smith (2000), in a Cochrane systematic review of four trials of therapeutic ultrasound involving 659 women, reported that based on two placebo controlled trials, women with acute perineal pain treated by active ultrasound were less likely to report no improvement (OR 0.37, 95% CI 0.19–0.69). One trial of ultrasound compared with electromagnetic therapy found those treated with ultrasound were less likely to have perineal pain at 10 days and 3 months (OR 0.43, 95% CI 0.22–0.84), although they were more likely to have bruising at 10 days (OR 1.64, 95% CI 1.04–2.60). One trial examined treatment for dyspareunia presenting at 6 weeks or later and found that this was more likely to be relieved after ultrasound than placebo, but fewer women in the ultrasound group had attempted intercourse. The reviewer concluded that there is not enough good quality evidence to evaluate adequately the effects of ultrasound in treating perineal pain and dyspareunia. However, in view of the potential benefit of ultrasound in general wound healing, the reviewer did suggest that further high quality trials were warranted.

Cushions and rings

Sometimes women are advised to ease perineal pain and discomfort by sitting on a rubber or sorbo ring, but there is little evidence of the effectiveness of these (Sleep 1995).

Pelvic floor exercises (PFE)

Sleep & Grant (1987) conducted a trial involving 1800 women to assess the effects of intensive compared with routine pelvic floor exercises on various outcomes, one of which was perineal discomfort, at 3 months postpartum. They found that significantly fewer women in the intensive PFE group (9%) reported experiencing perineal pain in the previous week than in the control group (13%), although there were no differences in the other outcomes of stress incontinence, dyspareunia or how early intercourse had been resumed. PFE are generally taught to prevent or treat stress incontinence, as described in guideline 5 on Urinary problems, but the findings of the above study suggest they may help relieve perineal pain.

Removal of suture material

No studies have assessed the impact on perineal pain of removing suture material either because the suture is 'tight' or because of friction from a knot in the material. Anecdotal experience, however, suggests that selective removal of material may reduce perineal discomfort.

Haematoma

A haematoma may occur following trauma to the perineum, inadequate suturing of perineal trauma or traumatic vaginal delivery including shoulder dystocia. Haematomas are rare among the postnatal population, one clinical review reporting an incidence of between 1 in 500 and 1 in 900 (Ridgway 1995). The site of the haematoma can be vulvar, vaginal or subperitoneal (Gross et al 1987). Onset can occur immediately following delivery, but delayed onset can occur days or even weeks after the birth, possibly a consequence of failure to recognise a haematoma prior to hospital discharge.

Haematomas are extremely painful and prompt identification and management are essential. Incision and drainage may be required to alleviate symptoms; however this will depend on the severity and extent of the haematoma (Propst & Thorp 1998). As this is an acute symptom, immediate referral should be made to the GP or obstetric unit.

Management: dyspareunia

There is much less research evidence on the management of postpartum dyspareunia. In the trial by Sleep & Grant (1987), described above, of routine versus intensive pelvic floor exercises, there was no difference in the reported prevalence of dyspareunia at 3 months. Nor was there any difference in subsequent dyspareunia or in the earlier resumption of intercourse between the groups in the trial of bath additives (Sleep & Grant 1988b).

Women who have had perineal trauma could be informed that they may find resumption of intercourse painful, as knowledge of this may provide reassurance that they are not abnormal. If women do find intercourse painful, lubricating gel may ease soreness on penetration, particularly when intercourse is first attempted. In the NCT survey by Greenshields & Hulme (1993), it was reported that some women found that vaginal lubrication, oils or gels rubbed into the perineum or relaxation techniques eased pain during intercourse. Women who are breastfeeding could be advised of this, as they may be more likely to experience vaginal dryness (Barrett et al 2000). Expert advice suggests that a specialist clinic can be of benefit in treatment of women who experience painful intercourse, although further research on the management of this problem after childbirth is required.

SUMMARY OF THE EVIDENCE USED IN THIS GUIDELINE

• Observational studies and data from trials have shown that short and longer term perineal pain and dyspareunia are common symptoms after childbirth.

• Evidence from various types of studies indicates that women who have instrumental deliveries have more perineal pain and dyspareunia than those who have other forms of delivery, but the independent effects of mode of delivery and type of perineal trauma are difficult to separate.

• Evidence from eight randomised controlled trials shows that restricted compared with liberal episiotomy policies do not differ in relation to perineal pain or dyspareunia outcomes but there are other adverse outcomes indicating that a routine episiotomy policy could not be supported.

• Evidence from four randomised controlled trials has shown that catgut compared with synthetic materials used to repair perineal trauma results in more short term perineal pain, although there is no difference in long term perineal pain or dyspareunia.

• Evidence from several randomised controlled trials has shown that the use of a continuous subcuticular suturing technique is associated with less short term pain than the use of interrupted stitches, but evidence on long term pain and dyspareunia is unclear.

• One large randomised controlled trial found a two stage procedure of perineal repair with the skin not sutured to be associated with a small reduction in dyspareunia at 3 months, although there was no difference in perineal pain. More research is required to assess the effects of non-suturing of perineal trauma.

• One large randomised controlled trial showed that vaginal delivery with 'hands on' compared with 'hands poised' was associated with less short term perineal pain but there were no longer term differences.

• Randomised controlled trials and observational studies of various treatments for postpartum perineal pain and dyspareunia show that evidence of long term benefit is poor.

WHAT TO DO

INITIAL ASSESSMENT

• Note delivery details. Observe perineum if possible, to obtain a 'baseline' recording. Bruising, oedema, inflammation or gaping in the wound edges should be noted.

• Examine the perineum to detect signs of possible infection, oedema or inadequate repair. Ask for description of type of pain (e.g. sharp or burning), whether it follows a particular activity (e.g. when micturating or defecating) and if there is offensive vaginal loss. This information may aid 'diagnosis' of the problem and enable more effective care/advice.

• If there is discomfort related to passing urine or frequency of micturition, exclude UTI (refer to guideline on Urinary problems). Check the woman's temperature. If she is pyrexial and pain is experienced during micturition, take an MSU and refer to GP.

• If there is a third degree tear, advice should be given on preventing constipation (refer to guideline 6 on Bowel problems).

• Following diagnosis of the problem, visits should be planned to assess progress once appropriate advice and/or treatment have been given.

Conditions which require immediate referral to GP

• Suspected perineal wound infection

• Suspected vulval haematoma (or referral to obstetrician, according to local policy).

PERINEAL PAIN

• If a perineal wound infection is suspected, a swab should be taken and **immediate referral made to the GP**. Ensure adequate analgesia and stress importance of hygiene to prevent spread of infection. A woman may also have complained of an offensive loss, which may be a result of an infected perineal wound. If offensive loss is reported but not associated with a wound infection, refer to guideline on Endometritis and Abnormal Bleeding for management of offensive lochia.

• If there is extended bruising and perineal skin is tense, shiny and hard, there may be a haematoma. **Immediate referral to the GP/obstetrician should be made**.

• Application of ice packs may provide short-term relief, but should only be used as a temporary measure as they may inhibit healing. Local applications which may be beneficial, such as 5% lignocaine spray or lignocaine gel, need to be prescribed by the GP. Further evidence is required of the benefit of the cooling gel pad.

• Regular analgesia (paracetamol) can be taken to relieve discomfort. If paracetamol is ineffective, referral to the GP should be made for a prescription for ibuprofen, particularly for women with a large tear or extended episiotomy. Medication that can cause constipation (i.e. cocodamol) should be avoided. Refer to 'Simple Pain Relief' section in guideline 3, for further advice.

• Some women find bathing soothing, but advise that bath additives will not aid healing.

• There is no trial evidence that alternative therapies have any effect, but anecdotal evidence suggests some women find benefit. Alternative remedies should only be used if the midwife or woman is experienced in their application.

- If a suture has become too tight and requires removal, this should be done with sterile scissors, not stitch cutters. The knot should be cut, not pulled through the skin. This may ease discomfort immediately and reduce associated swelling/oedema.

DYSPAREUNIA

- If the woman had any perineal trauma, observe (if possible) for signs of inadequate repair (sometimes trauma is not correctly anatomically approximated) or scarring of suture line, which could result in dyspareunia. If this is indicated, the woman should be advised and referred to her GP.

- If the woman reports painful intercourse, although there is a lack of research evidence on effective management, anecdotal evidence suggests use of a lubricant jelly may ease discomfort. This information is particularly important for breastfeeding women, who may be more likely to experience vaginal dryness.

- Anecdotal evidence is available on the benefit of oils and gels rubbed into the perineum to ease discomfort during intercourse, but these should only be recommended if the woman or the midwife has experience of using alternative therapies.

- Women who express anxieties about resuming sexual intercourse may be concerned about the possibility of another pregnancy. If so, contraception should be discussed and referral to the GP to decide on the most suitable method.

- If appropriate, discuss with the woman and/or her partner that enthusiasm for a sexual relationship may be reduced for a period of time after childbirth.

- If dyspareunia persists and the woman feels it is a problem, she should be referred to the GP.

GENERAL ADVICE

- Most women who have delivered vaginally will have some degree of perineal discomfort initially. Acknowledgement that perineal pain is common and that the trauma will heal in time, may help relieve any anxiety.

- Dietary advice to avoid constipation should be given, particularly if there is a large tear or extended episiotomy, as straining may increase perineal pain.

- Perineal hygiene should be discussed as appropriate.

- All women should be given advice about contraception and resumption of intercourse within 2–3 weeks of delivery, when some women will resume intercourse.

- Women who have had perineal trauma should be informed that intercourse may be painful at first, as this may reassure them that they are not 'abnormal'.

SUMMARY GUIDELINE

PERINEAL PAIN AND DYSPAREUNIA

INITIAL ASSESSMENT

- Obtain baseline observation of perineum to assess bruising, extent of trauma, healing and possibility of infection.
- If discomfort related to micturition, exclude UTI (guideline 5), and if third degree tear, refer to guideline 6 for advice on preventing constipation

IMMEDIATE REFERRAL TO THE GP IS REQUIRED IF:

- Suspected perineal wound infection.
- Suspected vulval haematoma (or referral to obstetrician according to local policy).

WHAT TO DO

PERINEAL PAIN

- If infection suspected, take swab and refer to GP.
- If bruising severe, exclude haematoma – if present refer to GP or obstetrician, according to local policy.
- Advise that ice packs or bathing may ease symptoms temporarily, but will not aid healing and ice pack may inhibit healing.
- Remove any tight sutures with sterile scissors as this may ease pain.
- Ensure nature of pain and exclude other possible causes, e.g. UTI.
- Anecdotal evidence suggests alternative remedies may be of benefit, but these should only be used if the woman or midwife are experienced in their application.
- Advice on analgesia (paracetamol in first instance) if needed. Consider referral to GP for ibuprofen or lidocaine (lignocaine) spray gel, according to severity.
- Review progress at subsequent visit(s).

DYSPAREUNIA

- Check for inadequate perineal repair, persistent perineal trauma or scarring. If persistent, refer to GP.
- Stress that use of lubricant gel may ease soreness on penetration.
- Ensure risk of pregnancy is not a concern and advise on contraception.
- Reassure that many couples find enthusiasm for intercourse reduced for a time after childbirth.

- **Refer to GP if perineal pain or dyspareunia continue to be a problem.**

GENERAL ADVICE

- Reassure that perineal pain is common.
- Give dietary advice to avoid constipation.
- Advise on perineal hygiene.
- Reassure that it is not abnormal for intercourse after childbirth to be uncomfortable and that lubricant gel may ease soreness.
- All women should be given advice on contraception and resumption of intercourse within 2–3 weeks of delivery.

REFERENCES

Banninger U, Buhrig H, Schreiner W E 1978 A comparison between chronic catgut and polyglycolic acid sutures in episiotomy repair. In: Kettle C, Johanson R B 2000a Continuous versus interrupted sutures for perineal repair. Cochrane Review 3. The Cochrane Library, Oxford

Barrett G, Pendry E, Peacock J et al 1998 Sexual function after childbirth: women's experiences, persistent morbidity and lack of professional recognition (letter). Br J Obstet Gynaecol 105: 243–244

Barrett G, Pendry E, Peacock J et al 2000 Women's sexual health after childbirth. Br J Obstet Gynaecol 107(2): 186–195

Binder A, Hodge G, Greenwood A M et al 1985 Is therapeutic ultrasound effective in the treatment of soft tissue lesions? BMJ 290: 512–514

Brown S, Lumley J 1998 Changing childbirth: lessons from an Australian survey of 1336 women. Br J Obstet Gynaecol 105(2): 143–155

Carroli G, Belizan J, Stamp G 2000 Episiotomy for vaginal birth. Cochrane Review 1. The Cochrane Library, Oxford

Dale A, Cornwell S 1994 The role of lavender oil in relieving perineal discomfort following childbirth: a blind randomized clinical trial. J Adv Nurs 19(1): 89–96

Glazener C M A 1997 Sexual function after childbirth: women's experiences, persistent morbidity and lack of professional recognition. Br J Obstet Gynaecol 104: 330–335

Glazener C M A 1998 Sexual function after childbirth (letter). Br J Obstet Gynaecol 105: 241–248

Glazener C M A, Abdalla M I, Stroud P et al 1995 Postnatal maternal morbidity: extent, causes, prevention and treatment. Br J Obstet Gynaecol 102: 282–287

Gordon B, Mackrodt C, Fern E et al 1998 The Ipswich Childbirth Study: 1 A randomised evaluation of two stage postpartum perineal repair leaving the skin unsutured. Br J Obstet Gynaecol 105(4): 435–440

Greenshields W, Hulme H 1993 The perineum in childbirth. A survey of women's experiences and midwives' practices. National Childbirth Trust, London

Gross S T, Shime J, Farine D 1987 Shoulder dystocia: predictors and outcome. A five year review. Am J Obstet Gynecol 156: 334–336

Harrison R F, Brennan M 1987 Evaluation of two local anaesthetic sprays for the relief of post-episiotomy pain. Curr Med Res Opin 10: 364–369

Hay-Smith E J C 2000 Therapeutic ultrasound for postpartum perineal pain and dyspareunia. Cochrane Review 3. The Cochrane Library, Oxford

Isager-Sally I, Legarth J, Jacobsen B et al 1986 Episiotomy repair—immediate and long term sequelae. A prospective randomised study of three different methods of repair. Br J Obstet Gynaecol 93: 420–425

Johanson R B, Rice C, Doyle M et al 1993 A randomised prospective study comparing the new vacuum extractor policy with forceps delivery. Br J Obstet Gynaecol 100: 524–530

Kettle C 1999 Perineal tears. Nursing Times Clinical Monographs 39. NT Books, London

Kettle C, Johanson R B 2000a Absorbable synthetic versus catgut suture material for perineal repair. Cochrane Review 3. The Cochrane Library, Oxford

Kettle C, Johanson R B 2000b Continuous versus interrupted sutures for perineal repair. Cochrane Review 3. The Cochrane Library, Oxford

Klein M C, Gauthier R J, Robbins J M et al 1994 Relationship of episiotomy to perineal trauma and morbidity, sexual dysfunction and pelvic floor relaxation. Am J Obstet Gynecol 171(3): 591–598

McCandlish R, Bowler U, van Asten H et al 1998 A randomised controlled trial of care of the perineum during second stage of normal labour. Br J Obstet Gynaecol 105(12): 1262–1272

Mahomed K, Grant A, Ashurst H et al 1989 The Southmead perineal suture study. A randomised comparison of suture materials and suturing techniques for repair of perineal trauma. Br J Obstet Gynaecol 96: 1272–1280

Moore W, James D K 1989 A random trial of three topical analgesic agents in the treatment of episiotomy pain following instrumental vaginal delivery. J Obstet Gynaecol 10: 35–39

Oxford Pain Internet Site 2001 http://www.jr2.ox.ac.uk/bandolier/booth/painpag/index.html

Propst A M, Thorp J M Jr 1998 Traumatic vulvar hematomas: conservative versus surgical management. Southern Med J 91(2): 144–146

Ramler D, Roberts J 1986 A comparison of cold and warm sitz baths for relief of postpartum perineal pain. JOGNN 15: 471–474

Ridgway L 1995 Puerperal emergency. Vaginal and vulvar haematomas. Obstet Gynecol Clin N Am 22(2): 275–282

Searles J A, Pring D W 1998 Effective analgesia following perineal injury during childbirth: a placebo controlled trial of prophylactic rectal diclofenac. Br J Obstet Gynaecol 105(6): 627–631

Sleep J 1995 Postnatal perineal care revisited. In: Alexander J, Levy V, Roch S (eds) Aspects of midwifery practice. A research based approach. Macmillan Press, London, ch 7

Sleep J, Grant A 1987 Pelvic floor exercises in postnatal care—the report of a randomised controlled trial to compare an intensive exercise regimen with the programme in current use. Midwifery 3: 158–164

Sleep J, Grant A 1988a The relief of perineal pain following childbirth: a survey of midwifery practice. Midwifery 4: 118–122

Sleep J, Grant A 1988b Effects of salt and savlon bath concentrate postpartum. Nursing Times 84(21): 55–57

Sleep J, Grant A, Garcia J et al 1984 West Berkshire perineal management trial. BMJ 289: 587–590

Steen M, Cooper K 1998 Cool therapy and perineal wounds. Too cool or not too cool? Br J Midwifery 6(9): 572–579

Yoong W C, Biervliet F, Nagrani R 1997 The prophylactic use of diclofenac (Voltarol) suppositories in perineal pain after episiotomy. A random allocation double-blind study. J Obstet Gynaecol 17(1): 39–41

3

Caesarean section wound care and pain relief

INTRODUCTION

In addition to the other changes of the postpartum period, women who have had their baby delivered by caesarean section have an abdominal wound which requires monitoring and care. In addition to wound infection other common infections following caesarean section include urinary tract infection (UTI) and endometritis (Leigh et al 1990). Urinary tract infection and endometritis are discussed in guideline 5 on Urinary problems and guideline 1 on Endometritis and abnormal bleeding respectively. The main issues in this guideline are wound infection and pain management.

The literature relating to wound care presented in this guideline refers specifically to caesarean section, but the principles of care can be applied to a postpartum sterilisation wound.

Caesarean section rates

The number of caesarean sections performed in the UK and other developed countries has increased steadily over the past 20 years (Savage & Francome 1993). A Department of Health statistical bulletin (1997) using maternity hospital episode statistics reported that 15.5% of all deliveries in England were by caesarean section during the period 1994–1995. This rate had increased from 10.4% in 1985. Another national survey of caesarean section rates found considerable variation between hospitals in England and Wales, with a range from 6.2 to 21.5% (Francome et al 1993). Savage & Francome (1993) found that women who attended teaching hospitals were more likely to have a caesarean section than women in other hospitals, but there was also variation in rates between teaching hospitals. Nice et al (1996) reported a range from 11.5 to 18.9% in five hospitals in West Yorkshire, the mean being 15.4%.

The trend towards earlier postnatal discharge from hospital for women delivered vaginally has also been seen following caesarean section. The average hospital stay following caesarean during the 6 year period up to 1994–1995 was between 4 and 5 days (Department of Health 1997), having been 8 days in a large national study conducted in 1983 (Moir-Bussy et al 1984). It is likely that all but the most immediate requirements for care of the wound will be in the community and more complications and infections will be diagnosed there (Beattie et al 1994).

WOUND INFECTION FOLLOWING CAESAREAN SECTION

Definition

There is no universally agreed definition of wound infection following caesarean section. Signs of inflammation such as erythema and induration are not specific to infection and irritation from the suture material can cause similar appearances. It is possible that serous discharge from the wound may occur without infection, but infection is likely when such discharge is purulent. Additional evidence of infection, in the form of positive bacteriological culture in material from the wound, is not always obtained. Studies vary in the criteria used to classify the wound as infected. The definition used in the *National survey of infection in hospitals* published in 1981 was that of inflammation or discharge of pus and positive bacteriological culture (Meers 1981). This was the definition used in a national survey of wound infection following caesarean section in 1984 (Moir-Bussy et al 1984). It was also the basis for the definition used in a prospective study following caesarean section by Parrott et al (1989), but in this study a wound swab or pus sample was taken for bacteriological culture from all patients with signs of wound infection *or* with postoperative pyrexia. A positive culture was accepted as evidence of wound infection with or without signs of inflammation or sepsis. In another study of post-caesarean women, the diagnosis was made on clinical features alone (Pirwany & Mahmood 1997). Leigh et al (1990) included cases with either clinical or bacteriological findings of infection. In one survey of general surgical patients follow-up extended into the community, and the definition of wound infection in a general surgery wound surveillance programme included cases where antibiotics were used to treat a previously uninfected but inflamed wound (Weigelt et al 1992).

Frequency of occurrence

Moir-Bussy et al (1984) undertook the first major prospective study of the incidence of wound infection after caesarean section in the UK. The method of selection of the 31 participating hospitals is not entirely clear so some reservations about generalisability of the findings remain. Survey questionnaires were completed for 2370 women having a section over a 12 week period in 1983. An overall infection rate of 6% (n = 141) was reported, with a range of 0–20.5% between hospitals. In the study definitions of classification terms used were clear, but there is no evidence that objectivity, consistency and completeness between and within centres were achieved. Indeed, although the definition of wound infection used was inflammation or sepsis *and* a positive bacteriological culture in material taken from the wound, not all centres involved in the study collected swabs for culture on all women with clinical signs. Culture from inflamed wounds was positive in 80% of cases and, in a later paper, the team suggest that if this rate were applied to the wounds recorded as inflamed but not cultured, the infection rate would have been 14% (Thompson et al 1987).

This study demonstrates the difficulty arising from the lack of a universal method of classifying wounds as infected when determining incidence of infection. Estimates of wound infection rates from studies which required positive bacteriological culture in the classification were: 4.1% (Hawrylyshyn et al 1981) and 7% (Hillan 1995). The rate was 11.3% from the study where wound infection was classified on positive culture with or without clinical evidence of inflammation or sepsis (Parrott et al 1989).

Higher rates were reported when clinical findings alone were taken as evidence of infection in the absence of a positive bacterial culture, with rates of between 15.8 and 29.2% (Henderson & Love 1995, Leigh et al 1990). The wound infection rate was 25.3% in Beattie et al's (1994) study which, in addition to clinical or bacteriological evidence, included cases where antibiotics were prescribed for wound infection without the study team having any further information of the clinical features. Follow-up in this study was also extended beyond discharge from hospital, which will further inflate the rate. In the report of a self-completion questionnaire survey at 3 months postpartum, of 444 women who had had a caesarean section 121 (27%) reported having had a wound infection at some point (Hillan 1992). It seems that for only 43 of these were antibiotics prescribed.

The trend is for rates to be higher when the diagnosis is made without requiring positive culture. Estimates based on positive culture alone are also subject to error. In the Moir-Bussy survey, *Staphylococcus albus* was the commonest organism cultured (Moir-Bussy et al 1984). The authors themselves acknowledge that this organism is an unlikely pathogen. If the cases where this was the sole organism cultured were removed from the numerator, the wound infection rate would have been 4.5% rather than 6%, but many of the cases where this was the sole organism cultured had clinical evidence of a wound infection. Classification for study purposes may differ from routine management, however, and in practice antibiotic therapy may well be instituted without culturing the pus or taking a swab of an inflamed wound.

As noted earlier, wound infection rates differed with time in Leigh et al's study of 202 women having caesarean sections in 1985 and 196 women in 1987 (Leigh et al 1990). All women in this observational study had their wounds assessed daily (excluding weekends) by the study laboratory nurse until discharge from hospital. Swabs were taken from all inflamed wounds, whether or not there was discharge from the wound. Wound infections were classified into two groups: clinical, where there was inflammation and discharge but culture did not show any pathogenic bacteria; and bacteriological, where recognised pathogens were present. The incidence of clinical wound infection was 20% in 1985 and 15.8% in 1987, but bacteriologically proven infections were 12.5% and 5.1% respectively. Since the same methodology was used for each series, with no significant difference in the caesarean section rate, it is surprising that the reported incidence of wound infection is so different. No explanations are offered by the authors. Other audits of different time periods have largely endeavoured to show an effect of antibiotic prophylaxis on infection rate (Nice et al 1996, Pirwany & Mahmood 1997).

Presentation

The onset of wound infection following caesarean section has been described between the first and fifteenth postoperative days, most commonly manifested on day 4 or 5 (Leigh et al 1990, Moir-Bussy et al 1984). Since some women will not develop the infection until after discharge from hospital, the true incidence of wound infection is probably even higher than that reported. The majority of studies of wound infection were hospital based retrospective chart reviews, leaving little scope for follow-up to identify infections after discharge. In almost all cases surveillance was limited to the hospital inpatient stay and although in one study observation was stated to be for 6 weeks, no indication was given of the completeness of hospital case notes regarding the period following discharge (Pirwany & Mahmood 1997). Hulton et al (1992) showed that the overall rates of infection following caesarean section were underestimates if based on inpatient data alone. They ascertained the infections which occurred following discharge by writing to the woman's surgeon at 6 weeks postpartum. The wound infection rate rose from 0.3% in 318 women who had caesarean sections in the 5 month period before this post-discharge method of ascertainment, to 3.9% in the 5 month period after it was initiated (n = 500).

Three studies identified women prospectively (Beattie et al 1994, Nice et al 1996, Parrott et al 1989), but in one surveillance was completed on day 6 post-section (Parrott et al 1989). Nice et al's study (1996) of 628 post-section women was prospective and follow-up was continued after discharge by the community midwife, but surveillance stopped at the tenth post-operative day. Beattie et al (1994) also identified 428 women prospectively and followed them up beyond hospital discharge but it is not stated for how long. Of the 83 wound infections diagnosed in the 328 women on whom the results are based, 30 (36.2%) were diagnosed after discharge from hospital.

It is likely, however, that findings from the Weigelt et al (1992) general surgical wound surveillance programme are paralleled for caesarean section patients. For 30 days after surgery the programme followed 16 453 consecutive patients operated on in various surgical specialties in Dallas, Texas, during a 6 year period between 1983 and 1989. Surveillance was by infections control practitioners (ICPs) and clinic nurses instructed in wound evaluation by the ICPs. Surgeons were not involved with the classification of wounds, to reduce any observer bias. Of all surgical wound infections that were diagnosed, 35% (516) first became apparent after discharge from hospital. Less than half (47%) of wound infections were manifest by the seventh postoperative day, 78% were diagnosed by day 14 and 90% by day 21. A small number of infections continued to be first diagnosed between days 21 and 30.

Of the wounds that did become infected, those which occurred in obese patients were more likely to be first diagnosed after discharge than in hospital.

As discussed previously there is no standard definition of what constitutes a wound infection, but the signs and symptoms suggestive of wound infection have been described above: pyrexia, localised pain and erythema, local oedema (induration), excess exudate, pus and offensive odour (Meers 1981, Morrison 1992). The diagnosis will therefore be made on the basis of patient reporting of pain, discharge, separation or fever and by visual inspection of the wound.

If a wound infection is suspected, a swab should be taken for identification of the organism and antibiotic sensitivity testing. The sample should be collected before the wound is cleaned, avoiding the surrounding skin, which may be colonised by different organisms from the one(s) causing the wound infection (Dealey 1994).

Apart from the need to relieve pain and dealing with discharge, the concern with any wound infection is the possibility of breakdown. Dehiscence (separation of the wound edges) may be superficial, involving only the skin layer, or may extend to the deep layers. In severe cases there may be protrusion of the abdominal cavity contents (burst abdomen).

Most caesarean sections are performed using a Pfannenstiel skin and lower uterine segment incisions. In a series of 1300 caesarean sections, the majority of which were performed through Pfannenstiel incisions, none dehisced although six cases of dehiscence occurred in the series following midline incisions (Donald 1979). Denominators for these figures were not quoted. Where the incision is midline, there is a greater risk of both dehiscence and herniation, but no published evidence of actual rates of occurrence following caesarean section were found. In abdominal laparotomy incisions in general surgical patients, the rate of burst abdomen (complete dehiscence) is of the order of 1–2% (Ausobsky et al 1985, Bucknall 1983).

Due to these concerns, women in whom wound infection is detected while they are inpatients are often kept under observation for longer. In the Moir-Bussy et al study (1984) average inpatient stay increased by 2 days for those who developed post-caesarean wound infection in hospital. The average stay for a woman who did not develop a wound infection in their study was 8 days. In the Canadian study by Henderson & Love (1995), the mean duration of hospital stay was increased in women with wound infection by 0.8 days in first section cases (from a mean of 5.9) and by 0.4 days in second or more sections (from a mean of 5.5 days) (Henderson & Love 1995). Mean stay was inflated more by certain other types of post-caesarean infection, but because of its relative frequency wound infection had the greatest overall impact on extra bed days required.

As stated earlier, follow-up data on caesarean section patients after discharge from hospital are scarce. Of 30 women in Beattie's survey who had a wound infection diagnosed after discharge from hospital, two required readmission (Beattie et al 1994). No details were given of subsequent treatment requirements.

Risk factors

In relation to *all* infectious morbidity following caesarean section (endometritis, urinary tract infection, wound infection, etc.), associations with many factors have been suggested (Hawrylyshyn et al 1981, Smaill & Hofmeyr 2000). There is less evidence relating to the risk factors specific to wound infection. There are no systematic reviews of the evidence and, as has been discussed, most of the studies are retrospective case note reviews relating only to complications identified during the inpatient period.

Using simple univariate comparisons between groups of patients in their survey, Moir-Bussy et al (1984) suggested that the following were statistically significant risk factors for wound infection following caesarean section: higher weight/height ratio (as recorded in early pregnancy); higher numbers of vaginal examinations during labour; longer duration of labour; not being nursed in a ward where only caesarean section patients were nursed; alcoholic chlorhexidine not being used for skin preparation preoperatively; the skin incision being paramedian or midline rather than

Pfannenstiel; having a drain of any sort; skin closure issues; having a plastic dressing rather than a material one; and being delivered by section in a unit where fewer than 50 caesarean sections were performed over the 12 week period of the survey (Moir-Bussy et al 1984).

Factors also considered in the Moir-Bussy et al (1984) survey, but found *not* to be statistically significant included: social class (proportionately more women from social classes IV and V were affected, but this difference was not statistically significant); emergency versus elective caesarean; duration of ruptured membranes; epidural or general anaesthesia; anaemia; and being delivered in a teaching or non-teaching hospital.

In their prospective study of 428 women who had a caesarean section, Beattie et al (1994) also described a link between obesity and wound infection, although they used last recorded weight as the index of obesity. Complete data were only available for 76.6% (n = 328) of the population in this study, and 44.2% of these women had some form of antibiotic prophylaxis. The study also showed a statistically significant negative association between maternal age and wound infection, but failed to show a statistically significant association between number of vaginal examinations and wound infection. Although there was a proportionately higher rate of infection for patients who had a drain inserted at the operation, this was not statistically significant. The authors state that a multivariate analysis method was used and the protective effect of prophylactic antibiotics was very strong so that demonstration of independent effects of other factors may be prohibited.

In general, studies have not attempted to clarify whether postoperative factors beyond the first day influence development of infection in the wound.

In a retrospective chart review of 1335 caesarean section cases between 1985 and 1988, Henderson & Love (1995) found that incisional wound infection was higher in first caesarean sections than in repeat sections, and was higher in elective section compared to emergency. Possible explanations suggested for this were decreased use of prophylactic antibiotics in elective sections, or that the interval between preoperative shaving and surgery in elective section may predispose to wound infection. Leigh et al (1990) found a higher rate of bacteriologically confirmed infections after elective caesarean section, but no difference for clinical infection.

Antibiotic prophylaxis

The evidence from 66 randomised controlled trials was examined in a systematic review undertaken to determine whether or not prophylactic antibiotic treatment given to women undergoing caesarean section decreased the incidence of febrile morbidity, wound and other infections or serious infectious complications (Smaill & Hofmeyr 2000). The review included trials that compared *any* prophylactic antibiotic regimen with placebo or no treatment. The lack of consistent application of a standard definition for wound infection (and endometritis) was noted in the background to the review and in the trials endometritis and wound infection were usually defined clinically—without bacteriological confirmation.

The main outcome measure reported was all infectious morbidity, and the findings of the review were that 'the use of prophylactic antibiotics at Caesarean section resulted in a major, clinically important and statistically significant decrease in the incidence of fever, endometritis, wound infection, urinary tract infection and serious infection after Caesarean section' (Smaill & Hofmeyr 2000). Only for endometritis was a measure of effect given, with its rate of occurrence reduced by 73% (95% CI 0.68–0.77) for all women undergoing the procedure. Prior to the review it was controversial whether prophylaxis should be reserved for cases where the risk of infection was higher, but the size of the reduction in endometritis was consistent even when elective and non-elective sections were considered separately.

Hospital stay was reduced by 0.34 days (95% CI 0.10–0.51) in those who received prophylaxis, but there was too little information in general to allow costs of the two strategies to be compared.

On the data from trials where elective caesarean sections were identified, no statistically significant reduction in wound or urinary tract infection was seen with prophylaxis in this group. Although this could be because the trials were too small, even collectively, to show a positive effect, the reviewers had to conclude that while prophylaxis is recommended based on the reduction in endometritis, the rate of wound infections following elective caesarean section may not fall.

The review recommended that all units should have a policy of administering prophylactic antibiotics at caesarean section. A policy of not treating all women undergoing caesarean should only be considered in units that have prospectively confirmed a low rate of infection in women using methods where follow-up was long enough to include late complications.

Another Cochrane review considered the relative effectiveness of different antibiotic regimens and found ampicillin and first generation cephalosporins to have similar effects in reducing postoperative endometritis, with no apparent advantage from more broad spectrum agents or from multiple dose regimens (Hopkins & Smaill 2000).

Management

There are no trials examining wound management in an obstetric population. However, a randomised trial of 1202 general surgery postoperative patients found that removing the dressing after the first 24 postoperative hours had several advantages (Chrintz et al 1989): wounds can be easily examined for early signs of complications; time and materials necessary for the renewal of wound dressings are reduced; personal hygiene is easier to carry out without a wound dressing. A sutured wound is not a contraindication to washing or showering after 24 hours. In this study there was no increase in the incidence of infection in wounds that were left uncovered after 24 hours. There will be circumstances when a dressing is required beyond this time, e.g. if there is exudate from a wound infection.

The aims of applying dressings to an infected wound are to absorb secretions and to protect the wound from injury and bacterial contamination. There is a wide variety of dressings available, making choice difficult. No single dressing is suitable for all wounds (Morrison 1992), and each wound should be assessed individually and comprehensively (Tallon 1996). Assessment should include the condition of the wound, the presence or absence of exudate, the depth of the wound, and the time available to visit the patient at home to dress the wound. The 'ideal' wound dressing is described as having the following properties: control of moisture content, gaseous permeability; no/low adherence; being impermeable to bacteria; thermal properties; protection of the wound from further trauma; being non-toxic and non-allergenic (Dealey 1994, Morrison 1992, Thomas 1990).

There is a lack of trial evidence to support any particular type of dressing specific to infected abdominal surgical wounds. Some health trusts have developed their own wound management policies.

No studies describing the indications for systemic antibiotics were found. In Hillan's self-completion survey of women post-caesarean section, approximately 7% of those who reported having had a wound infection had antibiotics prescribed for this infection (Hillan 1992). In women who develop a wound infection it is probably advisable to find out which specific antibiotic was given prophylactically, especially if treating them without bacteriological confirmation, as it may influence the choice of any antibiotic given.

Obesity is a risk factor for wound infection and, although there is no evidence of effective ways of improving risk, a higher index of suspicion should be retained in obese women post-caesarean. It is likely that women will be tentative in exposure of the wound when washing. Although there is no trial evidence to support the recommendation, it seems sensible to discuss the necessity, when washing, of raising any skin folds which occlude the wound when sitting or standing.

Adherence to correct hand washing techniques and general hygiene measures by health professionals and by the woman herself (Bell & Fenton 1993) is vital.

If surveillance is not continued until 21 days after surgery, the woman should be advised of the ongoing possibility of infection and whom she should contact with any problem.

PAIN RELIEF IN THE IMMEDIATE POSTOPERATIVE PERIOD

Wound pain

Few studies have described the occurrence of pain in the postpartum period. An Aberdeen survey of postnatal pain experienced by 198 postpartum women included 26 women delivered by caesarean section (Dewan et al 1993). The women were questioned about any pain—uterine cramps, perineal or abdominal wound, breast, etc.—experienced in the previous 12 hours. They were surveyed on days 1, 2 and 4 (if still in hospital). Overall, 95% of the women reported at least one type of pain on the first day after delivery, but by the fourth day most had settled. For the women who had had a caesarean the most important source of pain was their wound, and 73% still had wound pain on day 4.

The mainstay of analgesia in the immediate postoperative period has been opioid based drugs administered by injection. These may cause drowsiness, nausea and respiratory depression, thus reducing the woman's ability to care for her baby. Some trials comparing the efficacy of perioperative interventions in reducing pain after caesarean section have been reported.

Non-steroidal anti-inflammatory drugs (NSAIDs) have been used in the treatment of rheumatic disease for over 25 years, and during the past 10 years have become more commonly used to treat postoperative pain. Side effects are rare but the usual contraindications apply: bleeding disturbances, allergy or previous marked side effects to NSAIDs, asthma, previous gastrointestinal ulceration, atopia or diabetes, etc. Most NSAIDs do increase bleeding time slightly, and they may inhibit contractions of the pregnant uterus. Given in large doses NSAIDs can cause premature closure of the ductus arteriosus.

Publications on the use of NSAIDs in the relief of post-caesarean section pain have concentrated largely on the first 48 hours following surgery (Bush et al 1992, Dennis et al 1995, Rorarius et al 1993). Available papers, therefore, relate to relief of intense pain and the use of stronger NSAIDs, such as diclofenac. The measures of outcome often include whether the amount of opioid required—administered intramuscularly or via a patient controlled analgesia system (PCAS)—is reduced or delayed.

In a double blind randomised controlled trial Bush et al (1992) evaluated the use of a single dose of intramuscular diclofenac (an NSAID) after elective caesarean section under general anaesthesia. The outcome measure used was the patient's postoperative requirement for opioid analgesia (papaveretum) by a patient controlled analgesia (PCA) system. Mean opioid consumption in the diclofenac group was significantly lower than in the control group during the first 18 hours (61.4 mg vs 91.4 mg, $p<0.05$).

The authors also found that equal or superior analgesia was achieved within the first 6 hours with less sedation in the diclofenac group. This was a small study—23 women were allocated to receive diclofenac 75 mg, and 25 had an equal volume of normal saline—but the findings were consistent with previous work showing a similar effect following some forms of abdominal surgery (hysterectomy) though not others (cholecystectomy).

In a Finnish study, Rorarius et al (1993) compared the effects of intra-venous infusions of diclofenac 150 mg (n = 30) and ketoprofen 200 mg (n = 30) in a randomised controlled trial of 90 women who had elective cae-sarean section under spinal or epidural block. A control group (n = 30) received an infusion of normal saline. Requirement for postoperative opi-oids was decreased by 40% in women receiving NSAIDs. One of the women who received diclofenac developed uterine atony, requiring intra-venous uterine stimulants to be administered. It was the authors' view that the dosage of diclofenac received was insufficient to have caused this prob-lem, but the infusion was stopped as initial treatment failed to reverse the atonic uterus.

Rectal diclofenac 100 mg was assessed after elective caesarean section using spinal hyperbaric bupivacaine and spinal morphine in a double blind randomised placebo controlled trial (Dennis et al 1995). Women received either diclofenac (n = 25) or placebo (n = 25) suppository at the end of surgery. Subsequent postoperative pain relief was prescribed in accordance with local protocols. Observations including pain intensity were recorded at the end of surgery and at regular intervals postopera-tively during the first 48 hours. The mean time to first analgesia was sig-nificantly longer in women who received diclofenac compared with those who received placebo, but the additional analgesia required was similar in both groups. The authors attribute this to the efficacy of spinal mor-phine which meant that the overall scores for pain on mobilising was low in both groups. Although no serious atony was recorded in this study, side effects were recorded and whilst there were no statistically signifi-cant differences between groups, for two women in the diclofenac group the midwife recorded excessive lochia. The authors report that both these women had atonic uterus at caesarean section and before the diclofenac was given.

The numbers in these trials were small, the method of anaesthesia and postoperative analgesia protocols differed, and no systematic review has been done. While there may be some benefit from use of NSAIDs whether intravenous or rectal administration confers advantage over oral is not established (Oxford Pain Internet Site 2001). The need to record side effects is paramount for any future evaluations. This may be particularly important for those complications which, though rare, are peculiar to the postpartum period and may have serious consequences for the woman and her baby.

A systematic review of trials of incisional local anaesthesia for post-operative pain relief after various procedures at abdominal surgery showed that this method was effective for up to 7 hours in inguinal herniotomy. The effect was not, however, demonstrated following hysterectomy, though the studies combined still lacked the statistical power to determine whether there was an effect (Moiniche et al 1998). Caesarean section patients were not included in the review. There are therefore pitfalls in generalising findings from studies of general surgical patients.

From general surgical studies postoperative pain decreases rapidly to become negligible by the fourth day after surgery (Melzack et al 1987), but this will be influenced by any complications such as wound infection. Perception of pain levels differs between the patient and the nursing staff, with nurses more commonly tending to underestimate the patient's pain (Field 1996).

In most instances, however, it is likely that by the time a woman has been discharged from hospital after a caesarean section she will no longer require more than oral analgesia.

Simple pain relief

In Dewan et al's study (1993) of postpartum pain only 17% of the women treated with paracetamol and 58% of those treated with mefenamic acid (an NSAID) for postpartum pain had good pain relief. Whilst some drug combinations have been compared with single agents, trials of different agents or combinations are less plentiful. The results of such reviews and studies have been pooled with a single outcome—the number of patients needed to be treated (NNT) in order that one of them will receive a 50% reduction in pain compared with a placebo (Oxford Pain Internet Site 2000). Some reservation about the robustness of the resulting league table must be retained, as the comparisons are not made within the same randomisation and conditions may differ for the drugs 'appearing to compete'. As discussed, the comparison of analgesics is sensitive to pain intensity and the results which follow relate to moderate to severe postoperative pain.

Oral NSAIDs (ibuprofen, diclofenac) are most effective. There is no evidence that giving NSAIDs rectally or by injection confers an advantage. Injected opioids need to be given at higher dose to achieve an improvement on NSAIDs. The number needed to treat (NNT) for 10 mg of IM morphine was 2.9, i.e. for every 2.9 people treated, 1 will get a 50% reduction in pain attributable to the drug. The NNT to get the same outcome for ibuprofen 400 mg was lower and for diclofenac 50 mg was even lower—approximately 2.5. For paracetamol 1000 mg alone, the NNT was almost 5. The NNT for paracetamol 650 mg + 65 mg of dextropropoxyphene was slightly lower, but by adding 60 mg of codeine to the same dose of paracetamol the NNT was reduced to just over 3. With 60 mg of codeine added to 1000 mg of paracetamol the NNT was slightly lower even than that for diclofenac. The most common combined tablet in the United Kingdom is paracetamol 500 mg with only 8 mg of codeine. NNTs for this combination are not quoted and there appear to be no reported trials of the efficacy of this combination. It is likely that a reduced dose of codeine has less analgesic effect but a better safety profile. However, repeated doses may be more common if pain relief is less effective, and there may be cumulative effects as a result.

A standard prescribing policy would ensure postnatal women received appropriate pain management. Many women probably experience pain that could be alleviated, but because of failure by health professionals to acknowledge pain needs and apply consistent prescribing policies, effective care is not given. An example of a prescribing policy was presented in an audit of postoperative pain relief at home among 150 adults who attended a day surgery unit (Haynes et al 1995). Patients who underwent general surgery, ophthalmic, ENT or gynaecology procedures were asked to rate their pain as mild, moderate or severe at 24 and 72 hours and to record analgesia used during this period. Around half of the patients were managed according to the hospital's prescribing policy. Of 111 returns, 29 (26%) patients reported severe pain on at least one occasion and 12 (11%) contacted their GP or were readmitted because of poor pain control. As a result, the prescribing policy was revised—procedures were ordered according to whether mild, moderate or severe pain could be expected and prescribing policy amended to take account of this. A second audit of 200 patients over a 10 week period in 1994 found that 89% of patients received pain relief according to the prescribing policy and no patients had to contact their GP for postoperative pain relief.

The following prescribing policy is based on that presented by Haynes et al (1995), and it is likely to be appropriate for postnatal women:

- Mild pain—paracetamol 1000 mg four times daily
- Moderate pain—co-codamol 1 or 2 tablets four times a day
- Severe pain—co-codamol 1 or 2 tablets four times a day plus ibuprofen 500 mg twice a day.

Contraindications to NSAIDs should be taken into consideration: ibuprofen may be preferred to co-codamol in women where constipation as a possible side effect would accentuate perineal problems. Referral to the GP will be required for analgesics stronger than co-codamol and contraindications to NSAIDs should again be taken into consideration. The amount of NSAIDs excreted in breast milk is considered to be too small to be harmful (British National Formulary 2001).

SUMMARY OF THE EVIDENCE USED IN THIS GUIDELINE

- Midwives in the community will see an increasing number of women who have had a caesarean section, and at an earlier stage in their course.
- Lack of a single definition of wound infection makes evaluation of the evidence more difficult.
- Much of the data relating to complications following caesarean section are generated from retrospective case note review and confined to the woman's time in hospital, and there is little evidence of infection rates once in the community.
- Evidence from general surgery surveillance suggests that a substantial proportion of all wound infections will occur after the first week, though incidence falls after 21 days, by which time approximately 90% will have become manifest.
- There are no data on the effect of different community management factors (i.e. hygiene strategies, length and frequency of surveillance, etc.) on the occurrence or course of wound infection following section.
- There is evidence from systematic review that antibiotic prophylaxis is beneficial and it is recommended to all units on the basis of its efficacy in preventing endometritis. It will not eliminate wound infection completely and its influence on infections occurring later is not known.
- A strategy for the management of pain using paracetamol, co-codamol and ibuprofen may increase the number of women receiving effective pain relief.

WHAT TO DO

INITIAL ASSESSMENT—ALL WOMEN DELIVERED BY CAESAREAN SECTION

- Retain a high index of suspicion for wound infection, urinary tract infection and endometritis.
- Discuss with the woman the recovery from surgery and the potential risk of acquiring infection.
- Ask about general wellbeing, with particular regard to any signs of fever.
- Ask if she has received or is still taking any medication (antibiotics, analgesia). If taking antibiotics assess reason, and stress the need to complete the course as directed. If possible record whether antibiotic prophylaxis was used and if so which agent/s.
- Advise the woman on wound care. Tell her that wound dressings are not necessary after the first 24–48 hours if the wound is kept clean and dry.
- If the woman has had emergency surgery she may have a perineal wound as well. Check and if appropriate refer to guideline 2 on Perineal pain and dyspareunia for perineal care.
- Plan to remove clips or sutures when appropriate.
- Observe the wound and look for:
  — signs of dehiscence
  — separation of the wound edges
  — evidence of infection
  — tenderness around the wound
  — discharge from the wound: is it purulent? (i.e. pus)
  — redness spreading from the incision line
  — localised heat or swelling around the wound site.

PAIN RELIEF

- Pain relief requirements and options should be discussed with the woman.
- If the woman has effective analgesia from the hospital, this should be continued as prescribed.
- If inadequate, or no analgesia:
  — For mild to moderate pain suggest paracetamol as required up to 4 g a day in divided doses.
  — If insufficient on its own, or if woman reports severe pain, paracetamol may be used in combination tablets with codeine according to local midwives' prescribing policy.
  — If pain is severe consider referral to GP for ibuprofen.
- Review analgesic requirements and effectiveness at each subsequent visit.

DEHISCENCE SUSPECTED OR EVIDENT

- If wound dehiscence is severe, **immediate referral to GP or hospital should be made**. Explain to the woman and her partner that the GP may request hospital admission for assessment. If circumstances permit, apply sterile non-occlusive dressing.

- If bowel visible (i.e. burst abdomen) arrange immediate transfer to hospital. Apply a wet sterile pack or pad to the wound.
- If dehiscence is superficial, treat as 'evidence of infection detected'. If concerned, refer to GP immediately.

EVIDENCE OF INFECTION DETECTED

- Record the pulse and temperature.
- If wound is discharging or shows other signs of infection take swab, with sample of pus if possible, for culture.
- In dressing the wound it is recommended that local policy should be followed where available. If one is not available, a simple occlusive non-adherent dressing is best. If an occlusive dressing cannot be applied, the dressing should be secured with strapping to all edges to keep it secure.
- **Immediate GP referral** should be made so that the wound can be assessed, a specialist dressing prescribed, and any additional management instituted if appropriate.
- If sutures or clips in *situ* and enough time elapsed since surgery, it is common practice to remove alternate ones to allow drainage from the wound. If any concern regarding possible dehiscence, do not remove any clips or sutures and refer to GP.
- If pyrexial, advise paracetamol based analgesia unless contraindicated. Refer to GP if temperature exceeds 37.8°C and fails to settle after 24 hours.
- Look for other possible sources of infection, e.g. breast problems, respiratory tract, urinary tract, endometritis, perineal wound, and refer to the appropriate guideline.
- Reassure the woman and advise her to contact midwife if the symptoms worsen.
- Review as appropriate.

GENERAL ADVICE

- Take prescribed pain relief as necessary.
- If prescribed antibiotics complete the full course.
- Advise the woman to wear loose, comfortable clothes and cotton underwear.
- Give advice about finding a comfortable position for infant feeding (refer to guideline 4 on Breastfeeding issues).
- Take care of the wound:
    — bath or shower daily lifting skin folds if necessary to wash and (gently) dry the wound. If a flannel or washcloth is used it should be freshly laundered.
    — do not apply a dressing unless supplied by the doctor or midwife.

SUMMARY GUIDELINE

CAESAREAN SECTION WOUND CARE AND PAIN RELIEF

INITIAL ASSESSMENT—ALL WOMEN DELIVERED BY CAESAREAN SECTION

- Retain a high index of suspicion for wound infection, urinary tract infection and endometritis.
- Ask about wellbeing; any signs of fever.
- Determine current medication and reason for prescription.
- Assess the condition of the wound for: separation (dehiscence) of the wound edges; tenderness, discharge (type e.g. pus/serous); redness spreading from incision line; localised heat or swelling; odour.
- Discuss pain relief requirements and need for vigilance re. possible infection.
- Plan to remove sutures or clips when appropriate.

IMMEDIATE REFERRAL TO THE GP IS REQUIRED IF:

- Evidence of infection.
- Severe dehiscence.

WHAT TO TO

PAIN RELIEF

- Discuss pain relief and options available.
- For mild to moderate pain use paracetamol 1000 mg as required up to 4 times a day.
- If ineffective use paracetamol/codeine preparation or consider referral for ibuprofen.

DEHISCENCE SUSPECTED OR EVIDENT

- If dehiscence severe, immediate GP referral or hospital. Apply sterile, non-occlusive dressing if available – wet sterile pack or pad if bowel visible.
- Explain to woman and partner that GP may request hospital admission.
- If dehiscence superficial, treat as 'evidence of wound infection' but refer to GP if concerned.

EVIDENCE OF INFECTION DETECTED

- Record pulse and temperature.
- If there is exudate, take swab, apply simple occlusive dressing and refer to GP.
- If sutures or clips in situ, remove alternate ones if appropriate, unless signs of dehiscence.
- If pyrexial, advise paracetamol based analgesia unless contraindicated. Refer to GP if temperature over 37.8°C or fails to settle after 24 hours.
- Look for other possible sources of infection.
- Reassure and advise woman to contact midwife if the symptoms worsen.
- Review as appropriate.

GENERAL ADVICE

- Take prescribed pain relief as necessary.
- If prescribed anitbiotics complete the full course.
- Take care of the wound:
  — bath or shower daily lifting skin folds if necessary to wash and (gently) dry the wound
  — do not apply a dressing unless supplied by the doctor or midwife
- Wear loose clothing, use cotton underwear.
- Take care to find a comfortable position to feed the baby.

REFERENCES

Ausobsky J R, Evans M, Pollock A V 1985 Does mass closure of midline laparotomies stand the test of time? A randomised controlled clinical trial. Ann R Coll Surg Engl 67(3): 159–161

Beattie P G, Rings T R, Hunter M F et al 1994 Risk factors for wound infection following Caesarean section. Aust N Z J Obstet Gynaecol 34(4): 398–402

Bell F G, Fenton P A 1993 Early hospital discharge and cross infection. Lancet 342: 120

British National Formulary 2001 www.bnf.org/bnf/index.html

Bucknall T E 1983 Factors influencing wound complications: a clinical and experimental study. Ann R Coll Surg Engl 65(2): 71–77

Bush D J, Lyons G, Macdonald R 1992 Diclofenac for analgesia after Caesarean section. Anaesthesia 47: 1075–1077

Chrintz H, Vibits H, Cordtz T O et al 1989 Need for surgical wound dressing. Br J Surg 76: 204–205

Dealey C 1994 The care of wounds. Blackwell Scientific Publications, Oxford

Dennis A R, Leeson-Payne C G, Hobbs G J 1995 Analgesia after Caesarean section. The use of rectal diclofenac as an adjunct to spinal morphine. Anaesthesia 50: 297–299

Department of Health 1997 NHS maternity statistics, England 1989–90 to 1994–95. Statistical bulletin 1997/28

Dewan G, Glazener C, Tunstall M 1993 Postnatal pain: a neglected area. Br J Midwif 1(2): 63–66

Donald I 1979 Practical obstetric problems, 5th edn. Pitman Press, Bath

Field L 1996 Are nurses still underestimating patients' pain post operatively? Br J Nurs 5(13): 778–784

Francome C, Savage W D, Churchill H, Lewison H 1993 Caesarean birth in Britain. Middlesex University Press, London

Hawrylyshyn P A, Bernstein P, Papsin F R 1981 Risk factors associated with infection following caesarean section. Am J Obstet Gynecol 139: 294–298

Haynes T K, Evans D E, Roberts D 1995 The Journal of One-Day Surgery. Summer: 12–15

Henderson E, Love E J 1995 Incidence of hospital-acquired infections associated with caesarean section. J Hosp Infect 29: 245–255

Hillan E M 1992 Short-term morbidity associated with caesarean delivery. Birth 19: 190–194

Hillan E M 1995 Postoperative morbidity following Caesarean delivery. J Adv Nurs 22: 1035–1042

Hopkins L, Smaill F 2000 Antibiotic prophylaxis regimens and drugs for Caesarean section. Cochrane Review 3. The Cochrane Library, Oxford

Hulton L J, Olmsted R N, Treston-Aurand J, Craig C P 1992 Effect of postdischarge surveillance on rates of infectious complications after caesarean section. Am J Infect Control 20(4): 198–201

Leigh D A, Emmanuel F X S, Sedgwick J et al 1990 Post-operative urinary tract infection and wound infection in women undergoing Caesarean section: a comparison of two study periods in 1985 and 1987. J Hosp Infect 15: 107–116

Meers P D 1981 National survey of infection in hospitals. British Medical Journal Clinical Research Edition 282(6271): 1246

Melzack R, Abbott V, Zackon W et al 1987 Pain on a surgical ward: a survey of the duration and intensity of pain and the effectiveness of medication. Pain 29: 67–72

Moiniche S, Mikkelsen S, Wetterslev J et al 1998 A qualitative systematic review of incisional local anaesthesia for postoperative pain relief after abdominal operations. Br J Anaesth 81: 377–383

Moir-Bussy B R, Hutton R M, Thompson J R 1984 Wound infection after caesarean section. J Hosp Infect 5: 359–370

Morrison M J 1992 A colour guide to the nursing management of wounds. Wolfe, London

Nice C, Feeney A, Godwin P et al 1996 A prospective audit of wound infection rates after caesarean section in five West Yorkshire hospitals. J Hosp Infect 33: 55–61

Oxford Pain Internet Site 2001 http//www.jr2.ox.ac.uk/bandolier/booth/painpag/index.html

Parrott T, Evans A J, Lowes A et al 1989 Infection following caesarean section. J Hosp Infect 13: 349–354

Pirwany I R, Mahmood T 1997 Audit of infective morbidity following caesarean section at a district general hospital. Obstet Gynecol 17(5): 439–443

Rorarius M G, Suominen P, Baer G Á et al 1993 Diclofenac and ketoprofen for pain treatment after elective Caesarean section. Br J Anaesth 70(3): 293–297

Savage W, Francome C 1993 British caesarean section rates: have we reached a plateau? Br J Obstet Gynaecol 100: 493–496

Smaill F, Hofmeyr G J 2000 Antibiotic prophylaxis for Caesarean section. Cochrane Review 3. The Cochrane Library, Oxford

Tallon R W 1996 Wound care dressings. Nurs Manage 27(10): 68–70

Thomas S 1990 Wound dressings and wound management. The Pharmaceutical Press, London

Thompson J R, Hutton R M, Moir-Bussy B P 1987 Estimating the infection rate in mothers following caesarean section. J Hosp Infect 10: 138–144

Weigelt J A, Dryer D, Haley R W 1992 The necessity and efficiency of wound surveillance after discharge. Arch Surg 127(1): 77–82

Breastfeeding issues

Women need consistent advice on breastfeeding matters. In this guideline we have made every effort to ensure that advice is consistent with two important publications: *Successful breastfeeding* (Royal College of Midwives 1991), recommended by the college for all midwives to read; and *Bestfeeding* (Renfrew et al 2000), an international publication for breastfeeding women, from which material has been drawn.

INTRODUCTION

Breastfeeding has many health advantages for both mother and baby. Breast milk has been shown to protect babies against gastrointestinal, urinary, respiratory and middle ear infection (Howie et al 1990) and atopic disease if there is a family history of atopy (Burr et al 1989, Oddy et al 1999). Maternal benefits include reduced risk of premenopausal breast cancer and some forms of ovarian cancer (Department of Health 1994) and a possibility of protection against hip fractures in older age (Department of Health 1998). In addition, breastfeeding provides a unique maternal–infant contact and ready availability of food for the baby. The incidence of breastfeeding in the UK did not change significantly between 1980 (65%) and 1990 (63%) (Martin & Monk 1982, White et al 1992), although a small increase was reported in the 1995 survey *Infant feeding* (68%) (Foster et al 1997). Moreover, many women who start to breast feed revert to formula feeding within the first few weeks of delivery (Foster et al 1997), almost half within 6 weeks (Bick et al 1998, Department of Health 1995).

The Department of Health has estimated that the NHS could save £35 million each year in the treatment of babies with gastroenteritis alone if all babies were breast fed, representing a saving of £300 000 for the average health district (Department of Health 1995).

SUCCESSFUL BREASTFEEDING

Breastfeeding support should be seen as an integral part of the role of the midwife providing postnatal care. The Royal College of Midwives (RCM) publication *Successful breastfeeding* (RCM 1991), which aimed to make breastfeeding advice offered by midwives consistent and evidence based, stressed that this advice should be given equal priority with other aspects of care. The recommended duration of breastfeeding is at least 4–6 months to ensure that the infant receives the full protective benefits of breast milk (Department of Health 1994).

Almost all women who decide to breastfeed will have commenced this whilst in hospital, but most will now be discharged prior to the establishment of lactation, so that midwives in the community have an even greater role to play in breastfeeding advice. The World Health Organization (WHO) recommends that babies should have skin contact with their mothers within half an hour of delivery (WHO/UNICEF 1989). However a Cochrane systematic review of early versus delayed initiation of breastfeeding, including three studies and 209 women, found no differences in numbers of women continuing to breast feed (Renfrew & Lang 2000a), and not all babies will be ready to feed within the same time period. Babies have been shown to display a wide range of feeding behaviour following a spontaneous delivery (Henschel & Inch 1996, Widstrom et al 1990). Data from a national survey found that a longer time to first feed was associated with obstetric intervention, such as induction, caesarean section and the use of pethidine during labour (Rajan 1994). A Cochrane systematic review, including data from three trials, has shown that restricting breast feeds to a 4-hourly schedule (compared with more frequent or on demand) in the first few days in hospital is disadvantageous: restricted breastfeeding is associated with more complications and greater discontinuation of breastfeeding by 4–6 weeks (RR 1.53, 95% CI 1.08–2.15) (Renfrew & Lang 2000a). A high proportion of early breastfeeding problems may be due to incorrect positioning of the baby on the breast. A Cochrane systematic review, which included one small trial where breastfeeding technique was corrected, found that this reduced feeding problems and the likelihood of stopping feeding before 4 months (Renfrew & Lang 2000b).

The 1995 survey *Infant feeding* (Foster et al 1997) found that 12% of women who commenced breastfeeding gave up whilst still on the postnatal ward. It also found that being given formula milk whilst in hospital was associated with stopping breastfeeding within the first 2 weeks; 34% of mothers whose babies had been given a bottle in hospital stopped, compared with 11% where no bottle was given.

There have been various trials which have assessed the effects of postnatal support for mothers on the duration of breastfeeding. A Cochrane systematic review, including 13 trials of various types of extra support from professionals with special skills in breastfeeding, found that this resulted in fewer mothers stopping breastfeeding their babies within 2 months (RR 0.74, 95% CI 0.65–0.86) and fewer stopping exclusive breastfeeding within 2 months (RR 0.83, 95% CI 0.72–0.96) (Sikorski & Renfrew 2000).

Observational studies that have assessed decision making about infant feeding have consistently reported that younger women, those from lower socio-economic groups and those of younger age when leaving full time education are less likely to breastfeed (Bick et al 1998, Hally et al 1984). Since most studies have employed large scale quantitative techniques, subtle social and cultural influences that may affect decisions about infant feeding may not have been identified. A recent qualitative study of 21 women, which sought to improve understanding of how primiparae belonging to lower income groups had decided to feed their infants, suggested that breastfeeding is a skill which needs to be learnt, particularly by women with little exposure to other breastfeeding women (Hoddinott & Pill 1999). These authors suggest that women may benefit from an antenatal apprenticeship with a known breastfeeding mother. Low rates of breastfeeding over the past two decades means that many women may not have access within their social network to an effective role model.

A recently published cluster randomised controlled trial in Mexico City assessed the effects of home based peer counselling on the proportion of women exclusively breastfeeding at 3 months (Morrow et al 1999). 130 women participated; 44 received five visits, two in pregnancy and at 2, 4 and 8 weeks postpartum; 52 received one visit in pregnancy and two visits at 1 and 2 weeks postpartum; and 34 received usual care (controls). The home visits were made by peer counsellors recruited from within the same community, who had been trained by La Lèche League. Antenatal visits focused on the benefits of exclusive breastfeeding, the importance of positioning, and discussion of solutions to common breastfeeding problems. Postnatal visits focused on maternal concerns, information and social support. Both intervention groups were found to be significantly more likely to be exclusively breastfeeding at 3 months than the controls; this was practised by 28 (67%) of the six visit group, 25 (50%) of the three visit and 4 (12%) of the control group. These findings were not related to any of the socio-demographic, delivery or health factors examined. Further research, however, is necessary in other communities since findings may not be applicable across cultures.

Despite efforts to ensure that appropriate advice and support are given, there are frequent complaints from mothers of inconsistent advice from health care professionals about breastfeeding (Rajan 1993, RCM 1991). It is essential that professionals who have contact with breastfeeding women are regularly updated on breastfeeding matters. The Baby Friendly Initiative, a worldwide programme established by WHO/UNICEF, includes among its ten steps to successful breast feeding that staff are trained in the skills necessary to implement the policy (WHO/UNICEF 1989). A similar initiative for community based staff has recently been launched.

BREASTFEEDING PROBLEMS

It is likely that almost all postnatal breastfeeding problems can be prevented if the baby is able to feed effectively and efficiently from the beginning (Inch 1999). This does not always occur, however, so in addition to having knowledge about how to achieve effective, pain free breastfeeding, all midwives need to know how to manage breastfeeding problems.

Painful nipples

Painful nipples were reported by women in the 1995 OPCS survey of infant feeding as one of the main reasons for discontinuing breastfeeding (Foster et al 1997). Trauma can occur if appropriate positioning and attachment on the breast has not been adopted, as the strong suction exerted by the baby will soon damage the nipple. Unless a baby is correctly positioned and attached to feed, there will be little or no benefit from offering other advice, support and help. The Cochrane systematic review of feeding schedules in hospital, described earlier, showed that restricted feeding schedules whilst in hospital were associated with an increased incidence of sore or cracked nipples (RR 2.12, 95% CI 1.22–3.68) (Renfrew & Lang 2000a). Modern wound care management uses moisture (critical for epithelialisation across the surface of the wound) to aid healing. Hydrogel wound dressings to cover affected nipples have been used in the USA (Cable et al 1997). However, a randomised controlled trial in the USA which compared hydrogel moist wound dressings with breast shields and lanolin in the treatment of sore nipples found that although both treatments were effective when given with instruction in breastfeeding technique, significantly greater improvement was seen amongst women who used breast shields and lanolin (Brent et al 1998).

There is no scientific evidence to justify the use of creams, ointments or sprays to treat sore nipples. A randomised controlled trial, also in the USA, compared three topical agents to relieve nipple pain and enhance breastfeeding (Pugh et al 1996). The agents were lanolin, warm water compresses and expressed breast milk with air drying. All women also received information on breastfeeding technique. No significant differences were found among groups for pain intensity, pain effect or duration of breastfeeding. That none of the three topical agents was any more effective in relieving pain suggests that all three could be recommended to mothers, although creams may damage the skin's flora, which could lead to dermatitis (Renfrew et al 1990b). If women do want to apply moisture to their nipples, it may be more appropriate to recommend breast milk, which clearly has no side effects. One small study, which compared the effectiveness of a traditional nipple shield ('mexican hat') with a thin latex shield, found that the use of nipple shields only relieved symptoms temporarily and did not resolve the original cause of the problem (Woolridge et al 1980). More information is required to establish how many women continue to experience sore nipples, despite being informed of appropriate feeding techniques.

Engorgement

Engorgement results from venous congestion due to the increased blood supply to the breasts when the milk comes in. The volume of milk, if not removed as it is formed, will exceed the capacity of the alveoli to store it. Seepage of milk into the surrounding tissues will cause a reaction (because milk is a foreign protein) but not infection; women may experience pyrexia and tachycardia and breasts become red, tense, tender and full. Unrestricted early feeding and appropriate attachment of the baby at the breast are the most effective measures to prevent engorgement. The Cochrane systematic review of feeding schedules in hospital (Renfrew & Lang 2000a) found that restricted feeding in hospital was associated with an increased incidence of engorgement (RR 2.10, 95% CI 1.25–3.21).

Various treatments have been suggested to relieve engorgement if it does occur, but few studies have evaluated these. One recent non-randomised study compared one group of women who were encouraged to carry out prolonged feeding from one breast at each feed (n = 150), and a second group who were encouraged to allow the baby to feed from both breasts equally (n = 152) (Evans et al 1995). These researchers found significantly less engorgement in women who had carried out prolonged feeding from one breast at each feed.

Two early trials evaluated the benefits of manual expression of breast milk to relieve engorgement, and both failed to show any benefit (Inch & Renfrew 1989). Traditional remedies, such as the use of ice to reduce venous engorgement, or heat packs to stimulate milk flow, have not been evaluated (Enkin et al 2000). A small trial on the effect of placing cold cabbage leaves on engorged breasts at 72 hours postpartum found no effect on the relief of engorgement, and although slightly more women in the experimental group were still exclusively breastfeeding at 6 weeks, this was not statistically significant (Nikodem et al 1993).

Insufficient milk

A perceived inadequate supply of breast milk was the most common reason for cessation of breastfeeding from the first week until the end of 9 months after delivery, found in the 1995 OPCS survey of infant feeding (Foster et al 1997). Women may not be aware of the physiological processes of breastfeeding and, as a consequence, lack confidence in their ability to feed their infants. Advice from health professionals that might have helped women to overcome this may not have been offered or may have been inappropriate (Henschel & Inch 1996). It is difficult to obtain objective evidence of insufficient milk (Enkin et al 2000); however a very small minority of women may genuinely be unable to lactate adequately (Neifert et al 1986) and there is evidence from a prospective cohort study of 630 women of an association between postpartum anaemia in the immediate postnatal period and insufficient milk (Henley et al 1995). There are no randomised controlled trials of treatments for perceived or genuine milk insufficiency and research into this is urgently required.

Thrush

Painful nipples or acute breast pain may result from candidiasis infection (thrush). This can affect the nipples and areola and without treatment may spread to the rest of the breast or to both breasts; the infant might also have oral or perianal thrush. Thrush may occur when a mother has experienced no problems with breastfeeding, but has pain after a feed which can be severe and prolonged. The nipple and areola become red and inflamed and sensitive to touch. Women who have received antibiotics (for example prophylactic antibiotics for caesarean section or antibiotic treatment for mastitis) will be more at risk of developing thrush (Amir 1991). Treatment from the GP is required and some Candida organisms may be resistant to antifungal preparations. Nystatin suspension is usually prescribed for the baby and Canesten cream for the mother, but this needs to be washed off the breast prior to each feed. Expert opinion suggests that miconazole gel, which is an oral preparation available for use by babies, could be applied to the breast to treat the mother without the necessity of removal and, if applied before and after the feed, would also treat the baby. If local treatment fails, systemic treatment may be required (Renfrew et al 1990a), but evidence of the effectiveness of this is needed (Lawrence 1994).

Blocked milk duct

There is sometimes no obvious cause of a blocked duct, but it can occur as a result of incomplete emptying of a lobe due to ineffective positioning or attachment of the baby to feed, or pressure placed on the breast, for example from a badly fitting bra. As a result of the obstruction, the flow of milk builds up to form a hard lump, which the woman may report as being tender. In the absence of trial evidence, best practice recommends that the mother be shown how to position and attach the baby to feed, to ensure all areas of the breast are effectively drained, and how to gently 'massage' the lump towards the nipple when the baby is feeding, to aid the flow of milk (Henschel & Inch 1996).

Inverted or non-protractile nipples

Inverted or non-protractile nipples occur in about 7–10% of women (Alexander et al 1992), and women who have these may experience difficulties attaching their babies to the breast. It is the protractility of the surrounding tissue, rather than the shape of the nipple, that will determine a baby's ability to make an effective 'teat' from the breast (RCM 1991).

Antenatal treatments for inverted or non-protractile nipples have included the use of breast shells (Woolwich shells), Hoffman's exercises, surgery and a recently developed device called a 'Niplette'. Two randomised controlled trials examined Hoffman's exercises alone, breast shells alone, both breast shells and Hoffman's exercises and no treatment (Alexander et al 1992, MAIN Trial Collaborative Group 1994). The trials found no increase in breastfeeding duration in women who used either of the treatments separately, or both in combination. That flat or inverted nipples are not a contraindication to breastfeeding was shown in the MAIN trial, in which 45% of women with inverted or non-protractile nipples breast fed for at least 6 weeks, and women should be reassured by these findings (MAIN Trial Collaborative Group 1994). The 'Niplette' is a nipple mould placed over the nipple and areola. A syringe is used to apply suction to the device to draw out the nipple. There is currently only one paper that has described the use of this device in which the case histories of 14 women who went on to breastfeed following use of the 'Niplette' are reported (McGeorge 1994), but the device has not been subjected to clinical evaluation. If a woman is unable to initially breastfeed, expert opinion suggests that she will be able to express breast milk to feed her baby using a spoon or a cup (Renfrew et al 2000).

Mastitis

Mastitis is an inflammatory reaction to pressure placed on the breast, for example from restrictive clothing or ineffective emptying of the breast, or if a mother has missed feeds. It can be infective or non-infective, is usually painful and in most cases affects one breast. The prevalence of mastitis among breastfeeding women in the UK is unknown, but a prevalence of 20% has been reported in a recent Australian prospective cohort study, with most cases occurring within 7 weeks of delivery (Kinlay et al 1998). As a result of the difficulties in milk flow, milk collects in the alveoli, increasing the pressure. The resulting distension may be felt as a lump or lumpiness in the breast tissue. Even without infection, a substantial proportion of women may complain of flu-like symptoms.

If the pain and redness of mastitis do not resolve within 6–8 hours of either altering position to ensure effective feeding from the inflamed part of the breast or expressing breast milk to resolve the symptom, the mother must be referred to her GP, because of the risk of an abscess developing (Renfrew et al 1990b). An observational study from 30 years ago, of 53 women with a total of 71 episodes of mastitis, found that if treatment was delayed by 24 hours, women were more likely to develop an abscess (Deveraux 1969).

Breast abscess

The incidence of breast abscesses among breastfeeding women is unknown, but they are not considered to be a common problem (Renfrew et al 1990b). Standard treatment previously consisted of incision and drainage of the abscess as an inpatient, and regular monitoring of postoperative recovery. Dixon (1988) conducted a small study to determine if breast abscesses could be treated without an operation or readmission to hospital. Six breastfeeding women who developed a breast abscess within 3–6 weeks of delivery and had received antibiotics for 48 hours were included. Initially, pus was drained from the abscess using a 19 gauge syringe and needle, followed by a 7 day course of antibiotics. Aspiration was performed three times weekly until no further pus was drained. The women were reviewed 3 weeks after the final aspiration, by which time no symptoms of infection were present. Aspiration was recommended as first line treatment.

O'Hara et al (1996) carried out a retrospective review of the policy at Hull Royal Infirmary for the treatment of suspected breast abscess (ultrasound scan, aspiration of pus, antibiotics and repeat aspiration if necessary). Over a 2 year period, 53 patients were admitted to hospital with a suspected breast abscess; 22 were aspirated of which 19 resolved and 3 required subsequent incision and drainage. Eight patients underwent primary incision and drainage, one of whom required a second drainage. The abscess discharged spontaneously in five women. The remaining 18 patients had inflammation but no focal pus, which settled with antibiotic treatment in all but two. The authors confirmed that aspiration combined with ultrasound imaging was an effective alternative to incision and drainage.

WOMEN WHO REQUIRE ADDITIONAL BREASTFEEDING SUPPORT

Women who have a multiple birth

The advantages of breastfeeding for multiple birth infants are likely to be greater, since more of these infants will be premature and at greater risk of morbidity. Women who have a multiple pregnancy will require additional midwifery support and advice to ensure effective breastfeeding. It is very important to reassure women that the 'supply and demand' physiology of lactation means that they will be able to provide sufficient milk for their babies, even triplets. The evidence already referred to, on support and interventions to assist the establishment of successful breastfeeding, is applicable to multiple births. However, expert advice suggests that women may benefit from adopting a feeding routine, rather than relying on demand feeding, as this may make it easier to cope with the increased workload of looking after more than one baby. Further advice on breast-feeding multiples should be sought from the Multiple Births Association.

Women who wish to combine breastfeeding and employment

Between 1985 and 1990 there was an increase in the number of women who gave up breastfeeding within the first 4 months of delivery because they were returning to work (White et al 1992). This number has continued to rise, with 33% of those breastfeeding in 1995 giving up at 3–4 months because of employment commitments (Foster et al 1997). Several studies have found that a return to work is associated with early cessation of breastfeeding (Auerbach & Guss 1984, Barber-Madden et al 1987, Kearney & Cronenwett 1991, Simopoulos & Grave 1984, White et al 1992). An American study of middle class mothers found that those in part time employment breast fed their babies for longer than those in full time employment (Fein & Roe 1998).

A return to employment after having a baby should not be seen as a bar-rier to the continuation of breastfeeding, but women may need guidance on how to combine breastfeeding with employment. No studies have investi-gated the content or effects of such guidance.

INFANT CONDITIONS THAT MAY AFFECT BREASTFEEDING

Crying babies

A mother who is worried about her baby's crying may, as a result, doubt her ability to breastfeed and provide adequate nourishment for her baby. A mother may also be concerned that her baby has developed colic, a syn-drome characterised by paroxysmal, excessive and inconsolable crying (Crowcroft & Strachan 1997) and may link this with breastfeeding. Little is known about risk factors for the development of colic generally, nor the effect of feeding method. As part of a large study of infant health during the first month of life in Sheffield, information on colic was collected from the parents of 67 172 infants born between 1975 and 1988 (Crowcroft & Strachan 1997); 12 277 (18.3%) infants were classed by parents as 'colicky' some time during the first month. Bottle fed infants were less likely to be reported as colicky, but after taking account of the stronger relationships of maternal age, parity and socio-economic circumstances, the excess among breast fed infants, although still statistically significant was very much reduced (OR of breast compared with bottle feeding 1.09, 95% CI 1.02–1.15).

Few studies have examined ways of preventing or treating crying or colic in breast fed babies. Woolridge & Fisher (1988), in a review of the feed management of babies with colic, proposed that babies may suffer colic as a result of incorrect feed management, and being taken off the breast before receiving sufficient quantities of hind milk. As part of the trial by Evans et al (1995) referred to earlier, women were asked 6 months post delivery if their babies had colic (defined as episodes of inconsolable crying thought to be due to abdominal pain, and requiring medical advice). Of the 150 women in the group asked to carry out prolonged feeding from one breast, 19 (12%) reported colic, compared with 35 (23%) of the 152 women asked to feed from both breasts. Lucassen et al (1998) carried out a systematic review to evaluate the effectiveness of diets, drug treatments and behavioural interventions on infantile colic, with excessive crying or the presence of colic as the primary outcome measure; 27 trials fulfilled the inclusion criteria (interventions lasting at least 3 days in infants younger than 6 months who cried excessively). The results showed that elimination of cows' milk protein was effective when substituted by hypoallergenic formula milks, as was advice to reduce infant stimulation. The use of anticholinergic drugs showed some benefit, but due to reported side effects could not be recommended as treatment. A criticism of the review, however, is that the results of interventions in breast and bottle fed babies were pooled, rather than being presented separately, so no conclusions relating specifically to breast fed infants can be made.

There is insufficient research on ways to prevent or treat crying; for example to assess whether a change in feed management would reduce colic and stress in babies (Renfrew et al 2000b). Research into the effect of the mother's diet (including smoking and a high caffeine intake) and of non-pharmacological treatments, such as baby massage and support and education for parents, on a baby's crying is also required.

Weight loss

The RCM handbook *Successful breastfeeding* states that 'in practice, the simplest and most readily applied "yardstick" is that the baby should have regained his birthweight by 10 days of age' (RCM 1991, p. 34). However, this will obviously rely on an accurate recording of the birthweight. It is questionable, however, whether growth standards that were based on infants who had largely been formula fed should be applied to an exclusively breast fed baby (Whitehead & Paul 1985). A breast fed baby will initially grow more rapidly than a formula fed baby during the first 2–3 months, a rate of gain which slows down at around 4 months.

Jaundice

Physiological jaundice commonly presents in babies between 2 and 5 days old and as many as half of term babies develop this (Henschel & Inch 1996). Premature and/or low birthweight babies and those who are breast fed are more at risk. Breast fed babies tend to be at risk because human milk contains less vitamin K than formula milk (Canfield et al 1991). Schneider (1986), in a review of 12 studies, found a higher incidence of jaundice in breast fed than among bottle fed babies, but did not include details of when breastfeeding commenced or if babies were breast fed on demand. The British Paediatric Association (1992) recommends that all babies should receive a single dose of 0.5 mg vitamin K on the day of birth (orally, if this is appropriate). Breast fed babies require further doses at 7–10 days, 4–6 weeks and thereafter monthly whilst being exclusively breast fed. Concern was raised following the finding of a possible association between vitamin K prophylaxis and childhood cancers (Golding et al 1992). However, other studies have not confirmed this (Ansell et al 1996, von Kries et al 1996). Effective breastfeeding practices should resolve symptoms of jaundice but if the symptoms persist, biliary atresia should be excluded (Hey 1995).

SUMMARY OF THE EVIDENCE USED IN THIS GUIDELINE

- Evidence from a range of studies, including randomised controlled trials, has found that breast milk has many health advantages for the infant. Evidence of health advantages for the woman is less conclusive.
- Available evidence from a systematic review including numerous small trials of variable quality suggests that early support from professionals with special skills in breastfeeding results in increased duration of breastfeeding.
- There is evidence, from a systematic review of three randomised controlled trials of variable quality, to show that breastfeeding in the early days should not be restricted to 4-hourly schedules.
- Evidence from one large randomised controlled trial, judged to be of good quality, has shown that flat or inverted nipples are not a contraindication to breastfeeding.
- Trial evidence is available to show that sore nipples should not be treated with topical preparations. Further evidence is required to determine the most effective management of this and other breastfeeding problems.
- Available evidence from one small observational study and from a randomised controlled trial in Brazil suggests that women may benefit from peer support from a breastfeeding woman. Further culture-specific evidence is required of the effect of peer counselling on the duration and exclusivity of breastfeeding.

WHAT TO DO

GENERAL ADVICE FOR ALL BREASTFEEDING WOMEN

- The physiology of lactation should be briefly outlined, including the mechanism of milk removal from the breast and the composition of breast milk. Sensitively explore the woman's knowledge of breastfeeding: the advice received, key issues such as when to feed, how to avoid problems and if necessary deal with them.

- The midwife should ideally be present at a breastfeed to assist the woman to achieve good positioning (Fig. 4.1). However, if this is not possible the midwife could demonstrate different nursing positions, for example using a rolled up towel as 'baby'. Feeding positions include tucking the baby under one arm with his body curled around the mother's back. The mother would support the baby's neck and shoulders with the palm of her hand, her thumb and middle finger at the base of the baby's head. In this position the body of the baby could be moved towards the breast, thereby allowing free extension of the baby's head. Or the baby could be placed across the woman's lap with the baby's head and body facing her in one line. In this position she could use the opposite hand to support her baby as described above, or she could support the baby's head by resting it on her forearm (not the crook of her arm) with her hand on the baby's bottom, so enabling extension of the head.

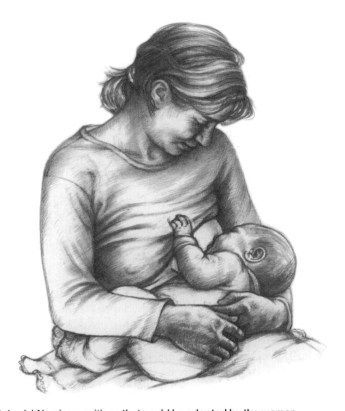

Figure 4.1 (a) Nursing positions that could be adopted by the woman.

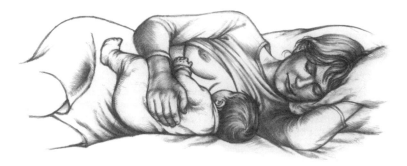

Figure 4.1 (b)

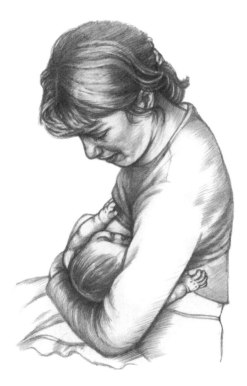

Figure 4.1 (c)

- When commencing a feed, the baby should be close to the woman, with his head and shoulders facing her breast and his nose at the same level as the nipple. The woman should allow the baby's top lip to touch the nipple until the baby gapes. The woman should then bring her baby quickly to the breast aiming his bottom lip as far as possible away from the nipple. The bottom lip will touch the breast first because the baby's head is extended (Fig. 4.2). This will ensure enough of the woman's breast is drawn into the baby's mouth to create a teat. When the baby commences suckling the woman may feel a strong 'drawing' sensation, but not sharp pain; the whole of the baby's lower jaw moves; she may hear the baby swallowing. A woman will be able to recognise if her baby is *nipple sucking* as she will feel pain; the baby will make frequent little sucks, will not change the rhythm of sucking and will not settle after a feed.

● If a feed is painful explain that this is probably due to the baby being incorrectly attached on the breast. The woman should gently take the baby off, then commence the feed again. Even if breast pain does not result in cessation of breastfeeding, discomfort can be considerable and last for many weeks. Appropriate and consistent midwifery advice can usually prevent or relieve this.

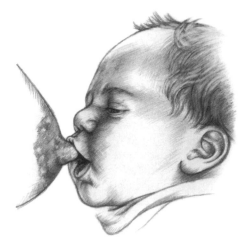

Figure 4.2 (a) How to ensure the baby achieves correct positioning and attachment on the breast.

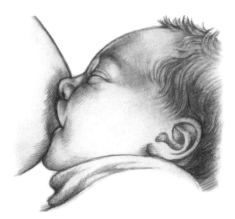

Figure 4.2 (b)

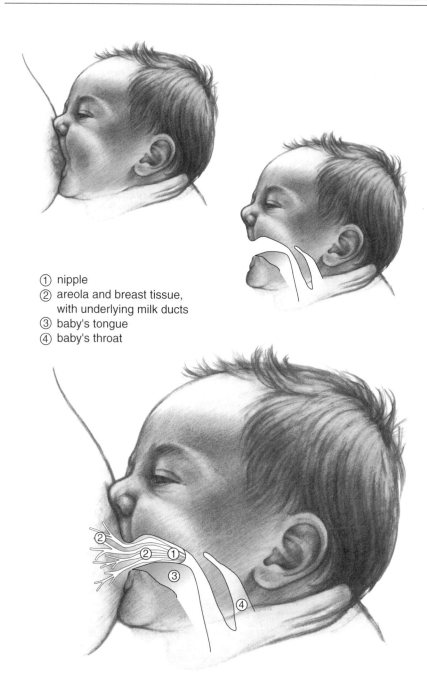

① nipple
② areola and breast tissue,
   with underlying milk ducts
③ baby's tongue
④ baby's throat

Figure 4.2 (c)

- A woman may initially need to support her breasts when positioning her baby to feed; once the baby is sucking, the support is usually no longer required, unless the woman has large breasts. A band of soft material loosely tied around the neck and looped under the breast could be used. Alternatively, she could support her breast by placing her fingers and palm of her hand underneath the breast, and gently place her thumb on top of the breast or back towards the axilla.

Other points of general advice are:

- Reassure that colostrum will totally meet the needs of the baby.

- Advise women that they may experience difficulties attaching the baby at the breast when lactation starts (refer to section on 'engorgement'). Reassure them that they can contact the midwife for help.

- Advise of the need for unrestricted feeding from one breast at a time when lactation commences, before feeding from the second breast, to ensure the baby receives both fore and hind milk.

- Explain that the baby will establish a sucking rhythm and does not need encouragement or stimulation to suck continuously. Feeding frequency may be variable, particularly during the first few weeks.

- Involve the partner and other relatives who may help to care for the baby in discussions about the benefits of breastfeeding and ways to prevent and resolve problems. Where the views of relatives are negative women may require additional midwifery support.

- Ensuring that all women have contact numbers for their midwives and local breastfeeding support groups will enable early assistance should a problem develop.

Expressing breast milk

There are situations when women may need to express breast milk, e.g. if they have engorged breasts, for freezing breast milk supplies before recommencing employment, or to involve their partner in feeding. If women can express milk and go out occasionally without their baby, it could facilitate longer duration of breastfeeding. There has been concern that if a breast fed baby takes milk from a bottle, he will not 'remember' how to take the milk from the breast (sometimes referred to as 'nipple confusion') but there is no evidence to support this. Women should be taught how to express, once lactation has commenced. Some women may prefer to hand express, others to use electric pumps.

Preparation. Some women may find initial attempts at expressing milk easiest in the bath or under a shower: warm flannels applied to the breasts may help to stimulate 'let down'.

Timing of expressing. The woman should express after a feed to generate 'extra' milk to store or to give to the baby later. If the baby usually only feeds from one breast, it may be helpful to express from the other breast at the same time, as lactation will be enhanced by the let down reflex. It is important to reassure that expressing breast milk will not decrease the supply for the baby, but will increase the overall supply of milk.

To hand express milk. Gentle pressure should be exerted on the inner edge of the ampullae, by placing the forefinger at the lower edge of the areola and thumb at the upper edge. Using a steady rhythmic movement, the breast should be 'massaged', ensuring all lobes are emptied in rotation. The woman may be able to express milk directly into a sterilised bottle where it can be stored for up to 24 hours in a fridge.

INITIAL ASSESSMENT

The purpose of this is to determine whether a woman is on course to breast feed effectively or already has a problem. *Appropriate positioning and attachment on the breast and unrestricted feeding will prevent and resolve most breastfeeding problems.* Establish breastfeeding history. The following checklist is helpful when assessing how breastfeeding is progressing. Check with the woman that her baby:

- sucks strongly and rhythmically, with occasional rests
- does not hurt her
- comes off the breast when he is ready
- during or after each feed, has the chance to wind.

The woman can be reassured from the following checklist that her breastfeeding is going well if her baby:

- grows steadily
- has straw coloured (pale yellow) or clear, odourless urine
- has a regular, soft (but not totally liquid) yellow stool
- breastfeeds well.

(Infant checklist, from Renfrew et al 2000, p. 83.)

Risk factors for potential breastfeeding problems (e.g. low birth weight and/or premature birth, multiple birth) should be considered when deciding upon the level of support a woman may require. Evidence relating to this initial assessment will also come from examination of the baby: jaundice +/–; hydrated +/–; drowsiness; weight gain.

At the end of this assessment the woman should be classed as on course to breast feed effectively, or experiencing problems.

On course to breast feed effectively as planned

- A woman says she is breastfeeding confidently, reports no breast problems, the baby finishes feeds spontaneously, is settling after feeds and physical examination of the baby suggests no problems. It is realistic, however, to advise that problems could still arise but these are manageable and should not necessitate stopping breastfeeding.

- Ask about breastfeeding goals: has she decided how long she will continue breastfeeding or decided to 'see how it goes'?

- Arrange an appropriate revisit. For example, if a woman is first seen prior to lactation it would be appropriate to return by day 5 to check there are no problems.

- At each visit encourage continuation of breastfeeding, ensuring consistent advice at all times.

Experiencing breastfeeding problems

- Obtain history: occurrence of problems in relation to feeding, woman's idea of cause.

- After discussion, examine the breasts, looking for nipple redness, cracks or bleeding, localised swelling of breasts, tenderness, redness. If she appears unwell take her temperature. If pyrexial, can this be related to a specific breast problem? Exclude other causes of infection and refer to the GP as appropriate.

After history and examination it should be possible to classify problems into the categories below.

Painful nipples

A sharp, acute pain when the baby latches onto the breast is likely to be due to painful nipples and is almost always the result of incorrect attachment. The woman may also experience nipple or breast pain when she is not breastfeeding. There may be nipple redness, cracks or bleeding but there should be no evidence of localised swelling, tenderness of the main breast or engorgement.

- Advice on the importance of effective positioning and attachment on the breast must be given.

- Advice on how to break suction gently with her forefinger when taking the baby off the breast may be helpful.

- There is no scientific evidence to support the use of creams, ointments or sprays or exposing the nipples to air, but they may provide temporary relief. It is probably better to advise the woman, if she wishes to apply some form of moisture, to rub expressed colostrum or breast milk on her nipples.

- Nipple shields are of limited value in resolving painful nipples, and should not be used before the woman has an established milk supply. If a woman is unable to feed because of severe nipple trauma, 'resting and expressing' over a 24 hour period may reduce the trauma (refer to Expressing breast milk, p. 74 for guidance on this).

- After 24 hours, the midwife should help the woman to recommence direct breastfeeding, ensuring that this is pain free. If the nipples are still painful, positioning and attachment should be checked again.

- The woman should be reassured that once positioning and attachment are effective, the nipples will heal very quickly.

Engorgement

This symptom is common when lactation commences, usually 2–3 days after delivery. Both breasts can be affected. Signs are red, tender and full breasts. There should be no signs of localised swelling. There may be a mild pyrexia, tachycardia and flu-like symptoms. Engorgement which occurs after this may result from the woman missing feeds, but the same advice should be given.

- Unrestricted feeding and effective positioning and attachment will prevent and/or relieve this.

- If the areola is engorged, the woman may need to be shown how to express sufficient milk to soften the areola to enable the baby to latch on (refer to Expressing breast milk, p. 74).

- Analgesia may be required (paracetamol should be recommended).

- Ensure that an obstruction in the breast is not caused by a badly fitting bra.

- Be aware that if engorgement is not relieved the woman may develop mastitis.

Insufficient milk

A woman may express concern that because her baby is not settling after a feed, is waking frequently for feeds or is not gaining weight, she is not providing adequate milk. This is one of the most commonly reported reasons for giving up breastfeeding.

- Reassure that this can almost always be dealt with since actual (rather than perceived) insufficient milk is extremely rare.

- Women should be aware of the importance of effective positioning and attachment on the breast to aid the establishment of lactation.

- Women should not limit the duration of feeds: the baby should empty the first breast before going to the second. After the milk is 'in' it is important that the baby is able to empty the breast of fore and hind milk at each feed.

- It may be helpful to suggest different feeding positions (*refer to p. 70*).

- If appropriate feeding practices do not alleviate the problem and there are concerns about the woman's milk supply and/or the baby's growth, referral to the GP should be made.

- Encourage and support the woman to continue breastfeeding. Do not recommend that the baby receives supplementary fluids until all efforts to establish breastfeeding have been made.

Thrush

The woman may complain of a burning sensation or deep breast pain, lasting for several minutes during or after a feed. The skin on the nipples and areolae may be red, itchy and shiny. There should be no evidence of localised swelling. The baby should be examined for signs of oral or perianal thrush. Immediate GP referral should be made for a prescription.

- Midwifery visits should be planned to check symptoms are responding.

- The woman may require pain relief when feeding, until antifungal treatments take effect.

- If symptoms do not respond in either woman or baby, or if recurrence is suspected, refer back to the GP.

- The woman should be advised about the need to wash her hands following each nappy change, to change breast pads frequently and to wear cotton underwear.

Blocked milk duct

The woman will be generally well, but will complain of a localised lump or tenderness, usually in one breast. This can occur at any time throughout the breastfeeding period.

- Advise on the importance of a well-fitting bra. Varying feeding positions may help to relieve the blocked duct (*refer to Initial assessment, p. 75*).

- Explain how to 'milk' the breast to relieve pressure on the blocked duct (*refer to the RCM's publication Successful breastfeeding (RCM 1991), p. 63*).

- Advise about the possibility of developing mastitis and the importance of adhering to primary intervention measures to avoid this.

- Visits to assess progress should be made. If a woman has a breast lump which does not resolve after appropriate management, she should be referred to her GP.

Inverted or non-protractile nipples

A woman with inverted or non-protractile nipples may experience difficulty achieving effective positioning of her baby on the breast, and will require skilled midwifery help.

- Reassure the woman that she is likely to achieve successful breastfeeding, as babies *breast* feed rather than *nipple* feed, but she will need more patience and help.

- The baby should be encouraged to take a large mouthful of breast tissue. The baby will help to draw the nipple out by sucking.

- It may help women to stimulate their nipples with their fingers, prior to a feed, to help them stand out.

- If, during the first few days after delivery, problems are experienced with direct breastfeeding, lactation may be initiated using a breast pump and the breast milk fed to the baby with a cup or a spoon. Once the milk is 'in' and the breasts have softened, further attempts at direct breastfeeding should be made. After a couple of weeks of the woman expressing breast milk, the baby is likely to be able to breastfeed successfully as the nipples may have been drawn out.

- If only one breast is affected, the woman could feed the baby from the unaffected breast and express milk from the other.

Mastitis (non-infective)

Mastitis commonly presents as a red, tender lump, usually in one breast. The woman may complain of flu-like symptoms and may have a history of blocked milk duct. She may or may not have a pyrexia.

- Advise the woman that she can take analgesia (paracetamol) prior to the feed to alleviate discomfort.

- The baby will need to feed from the affected breast first as the sucking of a hungry baby should encourage drainage. Frequent feeds will keep the breasts from becoming overly full.

- Ensure that the breast is emptied at each feed. If the woman has been unable to feed because of painful nipples, refer to relevant section for management.

- As with a blocked duct, the woman should gently massage lump (if present) whilst the baby is feeding to help relieve the pressure.

- Visit frequency should be discussed with the woman, but regular visits should be made to ensure that she is confident about her management of the symptom.

- Encourage bed rest and plenty of fluids until the flu-like symptoms have resolved.

- The woman should not stop breastfeeding, as this could exacerbate the symptom.

- If these measures do not ease symptoms within 6–8 hours, urgent GP referral must be made to prevent the possibility of mastitis infection and abscess; antibiotics will be required.

- Increased frequency of midwifery visits should be planned to give breastfeeding support and to observe the woman and baby for signs of thrush if antibiotics are taken.

Mastitis (infective)/breast abscess

The woman will report a history of sudden onset, flu-like symptoms and pyrexia. Cellulitis in a breast lobe or erythema around the areola may also be noted. The breast will be swollen, red and hot with intense localised pain. This may occur following ineffective or delayed treatment for mastitis or staphylococcal infection from a cracked nipple. If symptoms of mastitis are not treated, a breast abscess may develop.

- *Urgent GP referral is necessary.*

- A woman with infective mastitis will require antibiotics and analgesia, bed rest and plenty of fluids until flu-like symptoms have resolved.

- She should be advised to continue breastfeeding (providing there is no pus), or express the milk. The milk must not be left in the breast as, even with the use of antibiotics, an abscess could develop.

- If a breast abscess is suspected, it is likely that the woman will require referral to hospital when aspiration of the abscess will be undertaken as first line treatment, followed by a course of antibiotics.

- If pus is draining from the nipple, feeding could continue from the unaffected breast.

- Midwifery visits should be planned to ensure prescribed treatment regimen is effective and to offer support.

Women who may require additional breastfeeding support

Multiple births

At the initial home visit, reassurance should be given that the supply and demand physiology of lactation will enable the woman to provide sufficient milk for her infants.

- Practice suggests that the woman will benefit from adopting a regular feeding routine (not recommended for single infants), and if possible feed the infants at the same time, as this will enable her to rest. Feeding at the same time will also maintain prolactin levels.

- The woman may require additional advice on feeding positions.

- Contact number for local multiple birth support groups should be given.

Women who wish to combine breastfeeding with a return to work

Advice should be appropriate to the timing of the return to employment. Information on how to express and store breast milk is essential (refer to Expressing breast milk, p. 74). The National Childbirth Trust and La Lèche League provide advice on combining work and continuing breastfeeding but women need to know how to contact these groups.

- If a woman expresses milk during the early weeks of breastfeeding this can be frozen and stored in sterile containers with airtight tops.

- All stored milk should be labelled with date and time of collection. It can be stored in a fridge for up to 24 hours, or kept in a freezer for 6 months for term babies, and 3 months for pre-term babies.

- Although not evidence based, current practice is that any thawed milk should be discarded if unused or if it has been in contact with the baby's saliva.

- Women can express milk several times a day. Different methods of expressing milk can be attempted to find the most suitable.

Infant conditions that may affect breastfeeding

Crying

Women are likely to be anxious and find it difficult to cope with a baby who cries a lot. They may be concerned that the baby is hungry or has colic. However, it is difficult to distinguish these from other signs of distress in the baby.

- Observe the woman feeding to check that she has adopted an effective breastfeeding technique.
- Check that the baby feeds for long enough on the breast to take sufficient hind milk.
- Reassure that she will learn the difference between crying for a feed, and crying for another reason. Babies cry for other reasons, not just when they are hungry. A new baby will usually have a good feed if he is hungry.
- Ask the woman *when* the baby cries—if it happens after a good feed, the baby may have wind. Advise on how to wind the baby. She should check if the nappy needs changing.
- Calming music may soothe the baby, and walking in rhythm may help. If the baby does not stop, advise the woman to let him cry but cuddle him. Try to get the woman's partner or another relative to help.
- Ask if the woman has altered her diet as some foods may cause a reaction in the baby. If she smokes or has a high caffeine intake, advise her to cut down or stop as these could be causing a sensitivity in the baby.
- Before a feed the woman should try to calm herself, perhaps by asking her partner or relative/friend to take the baby for a few minutes. Reassure her that a baby who continues to cry for no apparent reason is just as likely to cry if he was bottle fed.
- If a baby continues to have episodes of inconsolable crying, but is otherwise healthy, it may be helpful to refer the woman to a voluntary support group such as CRYSIS.
- If there are any major concerns about the wellbeing of the baby or the woman, the midwife should consider immediate referral to the GP.

Weight loss

As a general rule the baby should have regained his birthweight by 10 days of age. Weight gain should be used as one of the indicators that the baby is healthy (*refer to infant checklist, Initial assessment, p. 75*).

- The baby should be weighed on the same scales throughout the postnatal period. Accurate information should be given to the woman, to avoid confusion. In the absence of trial evidence on weighing frequency, if there are concerns about the baby's weight and overall condition, weigh daily.
- The baby should be weighed naked, before a feed and at the same time of day, to minimise fluctuations.
- If weight gain is static or there is concern about weight loss, ensure the baby is effectively positioned on the breast and feeding duration is not limited. If a woman has no breastfeeding problems, she can be advised that she can supplement the occasional feed with a bottle, but only if lactation is established.
- If there is any concern about the baby's condition, taking other indicators of health into account, GP referral should be made.

Jaundice

Physiological jaundice may occur within 2–5 days of delivery. The baby's skin will have a yellow hue, he may be sleepy and mother is likely to report that baby is not feeding well. Stools may be green.

- Reassure that this symptom is common among breastfeeding babies.
- The baby should receive regular (at least 3-hourly) feeds.

- Arrange a visit to coincide with a feed to assist the woman in putting the baby to the breast. Ensure that the baby is well positioned to receive colostrum, which acts as a laxative and will help the baby to pass meconium.

- If the milk is 'in', emphasise the importance of the baby receiving hind milk, as the higher fat content is more effective at stimulating bowel evacuation.

- Fluid supplements should not be given.

- Blood should be taken for a serum bilirubin and paediatric referral made if symptoms are progressive and do not respond to effective breastfeeding practice.

- Every effort should be made to prevent separation of woman and baby if phototherapy is required.

- Ensure the baby receives vitamin K prophylaxis according to local protocol.

SUMMARY GUIDELINE

BREASTFEEDING ISSUES

INITIAL ASSESSMENT—ALL BREASTFEEDING WOMEN

- Evaluate breastfeeding
  - on course to feed effectively
  - problem already present
- Ask about the behaviour of the baby
- Assess knowledge and give general advice as appropriate

IMMEDIATE REFERRAL TO THE GP IS REQUIRED IF:

- Maternal or infant thrush
- Infective mastitis/breast abscess
- Major concern about baby's wellbeing

WHAT TO DO

PAINFUL NIPPLES

- Advise on effective positioning and attachment of baby on the breast
- No evidence that use of creams, ointments or sprays or nipple shields will resolve problem, but may give temporary relief
- Further visit(s) to review

ENGORGEMENT

- Unrestricted feeding will help relieve problem
- If areola engorged mother may need to express milk before a feed
- Pain relief (paracetamol) may be required
- If engorgement is not relieved the mother may develop mastitis
- Further visit(s) to review

INSUFFICIENT MILK

- Reassure that this can almost always be dealt with
- Discuss importance of positioning and attachment of baby on breast
- There should be no limit on the duration of feeds and emphasise importance of baby taking fore and hind milk
- If above do not solve problem and there is concern about baby's growth, refer to GP
- Do not recommend supplementary fluids until all breastfeeding efforts have failed

THRUSH/INFECTIVE MASTITIS/BREAST ABSCESS

- All need GP referral. Following this outcomes of treatment should be reviewed

BLOCKED MILK DUCT

- Discuss different feeding positions and check bra fitting
- Show mother how to 'milk' the duct
- Advise re possibility of developing mastitis
- Further visit(s) to review

INVERTED OR NON-PROTRACTILE NIPPLES

- Reassure mother that babies breast feed rather than 'nipple' feed
- If initial problems experienced with breastfeeding, initiate lactation with breast pump and feed baby with cup or spoon. Breast feed when milk is 'in'
- If only one breast is affected, feed from the unaffected side

NON-INFECTIVE MASTITIS

- Advise analgesia (paracetamol) prior to feed
- Feed from affected side first
- Frequent feeds ensuring breast emptied
- Gently massage lump (if present) whilst the baby is feeding
- Encourage bed rest, until flu-like symptoms have resolved
- Do not stop breastfeeding
- If symptoms not eased in 6–8 hours (telephone to find out), refer to GP
- If symptoms have eased, increase visit frequency until resolved

GENERAL ADVICE (FOR SUCCESSFUL BREASTFEEDING)

- Avoid conflicting advice
- Emphasise the importance of correct positioning and attachment of the baby at the breast — observe feed if possible, and describe lactation process
- Advise about different nursing positions; as long as correct positioning and attachment on the breast are achieved, no one position is better than another
- If suckling causes pain take the baby off the breast, reposition and reattach
- Reassure that colostrum will fully meet the needs of the baby, and complementary feeds are not necessary
- Emphasise the importance of unrestricted feeding on one breast, before starting the second
- Include partner and any close relatives involved in care of the baby in discussion of breastfeeding advantages
- If problem develops, midwife can be contacted
- Provide addresses/telephone numbers of local breastfeeding support groups

ADVICE ON HAND EXPRESSING BREAST MILK

- Advise the woman to practise hand expressing before stored supplies are required, for example before she recommences employment. As she becomes more confident, she may find other ways of expressing milk which she feels are better for her
- To hand express the woman should place her thumb flat on the upper edge of the areola and cup the rest of her hand under her breast. Her forefinger should rest on the lower edge of the areola. She should then gently squeeze her thumb and forefinger together, and at the same time gently press her whole hand back and in, towards the chest wall. Doing these movements together enables milk from the deep breast tissue to be expressed as well as the ducts beneath the areola and nipple

REFERENCES

Alexander J M, Grant A M, Campbell M J 1992 RCT of breast shells and Hoffman's exercises for inverted and non-protractile nipples. BMJ 304: 1030–1032

Amir L H 1991 Candida and the lactating breast: predisposing factors. J Hum Lactation 7: 171–181

Ansell P, Bull D, Roman E 1996 Childhood leukaemia and intramuscular vitamin K: findings from a case-control study. BMJ 313: 204–205

Auerbach K G, Guss E 1984 Maternal employment and breastfeeding. Am J Dis Child 138: 958–960

Barber-Madden R, Petschek M A, Pakter J 1987 Breast feeding and the working mother: barriers and intervention strategies. J Public Health Policy 8: 531–541

Bick D E, MacArthur C, Lancashire R 1998 What influences the uptake and early cessation of breast feeding? Midwifery 14: 242–247

Brent N, Rudy S J, Redd B et al 1998 Sore nipples in breast-feeding women: a clinical trial of wound dressings vs conventional care. Arch Pediatr Adolesc Med 152(11): 1077–1082

British Paediatric Association 1992 Vitamin K prophylaxis in infancy: report of an expert committee funded by the Department of Child Health. BPA, London

Burr M L, Miskelly F G, Butland B K et al 1989 Environmental factors and symptoms in infants at high risk of allergy. J Epidemiol Community Health 43: 125–132

Cable B, Stewart M, Davis J 1997 Nipple wound care: a new approach to an old problem. J Hum Lactation 13(4): 313–318

Canfield L M, Hopkinson J M, Lima A F et al 1991 Vitamin K in colostrum and mature human milk over the lactation period—a cross sectional study. Am J Clin Nutr 53: 730–735

Crowcroft N S, Strachan D P 1997 The social origins of infantile colic: questionnaire study covering 76 747 infants. BMJ 314: 1325–1328

Department of Health 1994 Weaning and the weaning diet. The Stationery Office, London

Department of Health 1995 Breastfeeding: good practice guidance to the NHS. HMSO, London

Department of Health 1998 Department of Health, Nutrition and Bone Health COMA Expert Group. Report on health and social subjects 49. The Stationery Office, London

Deveraux W P 1969 Acute puerperal mastitis. Evaluation of its management. Am J Obstet Gynecol 108(1): 78–81

Dixon J M 1988 Repeated aspiration of breast abscesses in lactating women. BMJ 297: 1517–1518

Enkin M, Keirse M J N C, Renfrew M et al 2000 A guide to effective care in pregnancy and childbirth, 3rd edn. Oxford University Press, Oxford

Evans K, Evans R, Simmer K 1995 Effect of the method of breast feeding on breast engorgement, mastitis and infantile colic. Acta Paediatr 84(8): 849–852

Fein S B, Roe B 1998 The effect of work status on initiation and duration of breastfeeding. Am J Public Health 88: 1042–1046

Foster K, Lader D, Cheesbrough S 1997 Infant feeding 1995. The Stationery Office, London

Golding J, Greenwood R, Birmingham K et al 1992 Childhood cancer, intramuscular vitamin K and pethidine given in labour. BMJ 305: 341–346

Hally M R, Bond J, Crawley J et al 1984 Factors influencing the feeding of first born infants. Acta Paediatr 73: 33–39

Henley S J, Anderson C M, Avery M D et al 1995 Anemia and insufficient milk in first-time mothers. Birth 22(2): 87–92

Henschel D, Inch S 1996 Breastfeeding: a guide for midwives. Books for Midwives Press, Hale, Cheshire

Hey E 1995 Neonatal jaundice—how much do we really know? MIDIRS Midwifery Digest 5(1): 4–8

Hoddinott P, Pill R 1999 Qualitative study of decisions about infant feeding among women in east end of London. BMJ 318: 30–34

Howie P W, Forsyth J S, Ogston S A et al 1990 Protective effect of breast feeding against infection. BMJ 300: 11–16

Inch S 1999 Breast feeding update. In: Alexander J, Roth C, Levy V (eds) Midwifery practice. Core topics 3. Macmillan Press, Basingstoke

Inch S, Fisher C 1999 Breast feeding. In: Marsh G, Renfrew M (eds) Community-based maternity care. Oxford University Press, Oxford

Inch S, Renfrew M 1989 Common breastfeeding problems. In: Chalmers I, Enkin M, Keirse M (eds) Effective care in pregnancy and childbirth. Oxford University Press, Oxford

Kearney M H, Cronenwett L 1991 Breast feeding and employment. J Gynaecol Neonatal Nurs 20: 471–480

Kinlay J R, O'Connell D L, Kinlay S 1998 Incidence of mastitis in breastfeeding women six months after delivery: a prospective cohort study. Med J Aust 169(6): 310–312

Lawrence R 1994 Breastfeeding – a guide for the medical profession, 4th edn. Mosby Company, New York

Lucassen P L B J, Assendelft W J J, Gubbels J W et al 1998 Effectiveness of treatments for infantile colic: systematic review. BMJ 316: 1563–1569

McGeorge D D 1994 The 'Niplette': an instrument for the non-surgical correction of inverted nipples. Br J Plast Surg 47(1): 46–49

MAIN Trial Collaborative Group 1994 Preparing for breast feeding: treatment of inverted and non-protractile nipples in pregnancy. Midwifery 10(4): 200–214

Martin J, Monk J 1982 Infant feeding 1980. HMSO, London

Morrow A L, Guerrero M L, Shults J et al 1999 Efficacy of home-based peer counselling to promote exclusive breastfeeding: a randomised controlled trial. Lancet 353(9160): 1226–1231

Neifert M R, Seacat J M, Jobe W E 1986 Lactation failure due to insufficient glandular development of the breast. Pediatrics 76: 823–828

Nikodem V C, Danzinger D, Gebka N et al 1993 Do cabbage leaves prevent engorgement? A randomised controlled study. Birth 20: 61–64

Oddy W H, Holt P G, Sly P D et al 1999 Association between breast feeding and asthma in 6 year old children: findings of a prospective birth cohort study. BMJ 319: 815–819

O'Hara R J, Dexter S P, Fox J N 1996 Conservative management of infective mastitis and breast abscesses after ultrasonographic assessment. Brit J Surg 83(10): 1413–1414

Pugh L C, Buchko B L, Bishop B A et al 1996 A comparison of topical agents to relieve nipple pain and enhance breastfeeding. Birth 23(2): 88–93

Rajan L 1993 The contribution of professional support, information and consistent advice to successful breast feeding. Midwifery 9: 197–209

Rajan L 1994 The impact of obstetric procedures and analgesia/anaesthesia during labour and delivery on breast feeding. Midwifery 10: 87–103

Renfrew M J, Lang S 2000a Feeding schedules in hospitals for newborn infants. Cochrane Review 3. The Cochrane Library, Oxford

Renfrew M J, Lang S 2000b Interventions for improving breastfeeding technique. Cochrane Review 3: The Cochrane Library, Oxford

Renfrew M, Fisher C, Arms S 2000 The new Bestfeeding: getting breastfeeding right for you, 2nd edn. Celestial Arts, Berkeley, California

Renfrew M J, Woolridge M, Ross McGill H 2000b Enabling women to breast feed. A structured review of the evidence. The Stationery Office, London

Royal College of Midwives 1991 Successful breastfeeding, 2nd edn. Churchill Livingstone, Edinburgh

Schneider A P 1986 Breast milk and jaundice in the newborn—a real entity. JAMA 225: 3270–3274

Sikorski J, Renfrew M J 2000 Support for breastfeeding mothers. Cochrane Review 3. The Cochrane Library, Oxford

Simopoulos A P, Grave G D 1984 Factors associated with the choice and duration of infant feeding practice. Pediatrics 74(4): 603–614

Von Kries R, Gobel O, Machmeister A et al 1996 Vitamin K and childhood cancer: a population based case-control study in Lower Saxony, Germany. BMJ 313: 199–203

White A, Freeth S, O'Brien M 1992 Infant feeding 1990. A survey carried out for the DHSS by the Office of Population Censuses and Surveys. HMSO, London

Whitehead R G, Paul A A 1985 Growth charts and the assessment of infant feeding practices in the western world and in developing countries. Early Hum Dev 9: 187–207

WHO/UNICEF 1989 UK baby friendly initiative self appraisal tool. UK Baby Friendly Initiative, London

Widstrom A M, Wahlberg V, Matthiesen A et al 1990 Short-term effects of early sucking and touch of the nipple on maternal behaviour. Early Hum Dev 21: 153–163

Woolridge M W, Fisher C 1988 Colic 'overfeeding' and symptoms of lactose malabsorption in the breastfed baby: a possible artifact of feed management? Lancet 2: 382–384

Woolridge M W, Baum D, Drewett R F 1980 Effect of traditional and of a new nipple shield on sucking patterns and milk flow. Early Hum Dev 4(4): 357–364

5

Urinary problems

INTRODUCTION

Symptoms of stress incontinence are the most common of the urinary problems that occur in pregnancy and the puerperium. Urinary tract infection (UTI), detrusor instability (including urge incontinence), urinary retention and voiding difficulties and fistulae can also occur, although the latter is rarely diagnosed among postnatal women in developed countries. All are reviewed in this guideline.

STRESS INCONTINENCE
Definition

There is some confusion surrounding the term 'stress incontinence'. It can be used either to describe a symptom or as a medical diagnosis. When describing a symptom it refers to the involuntary leakage of urine, usually on exertion. As a diagnosis it refers to involuntary loss of urine when the intravesical pressure exceeds that of the urethra, with no simultaneous detrusor contraction (Abrams et al 1990). The International Continence Society refers to the latter as 'genuine stress incontinence', but it is considered that this diagnosis should only be made following urodynamic investigation (Cardozo & Khullar 1995). The definition of stress incontinence used in this guideline, unless otherwise specified, refers to a symptom rather than a diagnosis.

Frequency of occurrence

The prevalence of stress incontinence in the general female population varies according to the definition used, and the age groups included, but it is very common and is much more common in women than in men (Burgio et al 1991, Holst & Wilson 1988, O'Brien et al 1991, Yarnell et al 1981). Several observational studies have examined the prevalence of urinary incontinence in postpartum women, again with variations in prevalence according to the definition used. In an observational study of 1505 women in New Zealand, 23.9% reported, by postal questionnaire at 3 months, some degree of urinary stress incontinence (Wilson et al 1996). (A further 10.4% reported symptoms of urge incontinence—see p. 95.) A UK questionnaire survey of 11 701 women contacted 1–9 years after birth found that 15.2% reported new stress incontinence that had started for the first time within 3 months of the delivery and lasted beyond 6 weeks (MacArthur et al 1991). A further 5.4% reported a similar duration of stress incontinence, but they had also experienced the symptom previously, either during or prior to pregnancy.

In an Australian study of 1336 women sent postal questionnaires at 6–7 months postpartum, a prevalence of stress incontinence of 11% was found (Brown & Lumley 1998). This was lower than that found in other studies, but the wording of the questionnaire was whether the stress incontinence had been 'a problem' for them, and there is evidence to suggest that postpartum women do not always consider stress incontinence to be a problem.

Some studies have documented that stress incontinence can persist for months or even years after childbirth. Sleep & Grant (1987a), in following up the population of a trial of perineal management regimens (see guideline 2 on Perineal pain and dyspareunia), found a similar prevalence of stress incontinence at the 3 year follow-up (23%) as at the 3 month follow-up (Sleep et al 1984). MacArthur et al (1991) found that among the 15.2% of women who had new stress incontinence after giving birth, three quarters still had this 1 year later. A recent European longitudinal survey of health problems among women at 5 and 12 months after birth found 1.7% of women in Italy and 7.6% in France reported urinary incontinence at 5 months. At the 12 month follow-up, this symptom was reported by 5.0% and 14% of women respectively. The prevalences were lower than in other studies but in both countries there was an increase over time (Saurel-Cubizolles et al 2000).

Severity reports of postpartum stress incontinence are variable. Bick & MacArthur (1995), in a questionnaire survey of 1278 women at 6–7 months postpartum, assessed symptom severity (average rating on a 100 mm visual analogue scale was 28.2). Most women did not rate stress incontinence as severe, although in answer to another question, 47% of the symptomatic women reported having to wear pads at some time to protect against involuntary leakage of urine. In the study by Wilson et al (1996), 129 (25%) of the 516 women with urinary incontinence reported using pads. Many women were found to view stress incontinence as an expected consequence of childbirth (Bick & MacArthur 1995). Nevertheless, it has been shown that some report that this symptom does have an effect on their lifestyles, including both physical and psychological effects (Mason et al 1999).

Risk factors

Although childbirth is generally considered to be a major cause of stress incontinence, and general population studies show it to be more frequent in parous than nulliparous women (Assassa et al 2000, Jolleys 1988, Thomas et al 1980, Yarnell et al 1981, 1982), the precise causative roles of the various factors are still not fully understood. Obstetric factors have been examined in both epidemiological and urodynamic studies. Caesarean section, whether performed electively or during labour, has been found to be associated with less stress incontinence (Assassa et al 2000, Dimpfl et al 1992, MacArthur et al 1991, Wilson et al 1996), which is consistent with findings of urodynamic investigations of pelvic floor damage (Snooks et al 1986). Wilson et al (1996), however, found this applied only to women who had one or two caesarean sections: women having more than two were found to have a similar prevalence of incontinence to those having vaginal delivery.

Urodynamic investigations have consistently found pelvic floor damage to be more common after a longer second stage labour and the delivery of a bigger baby, but findings relating to forceps delivery have been inconsistent (Allen et al 1990, Meyer et al 1998, Snooks et al 1984, 1986). In the surveys by MacArthur et al (1991) and Brown & Lumley (1998), stress incontinence was found to be more common after forceps delivery and longer second stage labour. However, the two are closely interrelated and the effect of forceps disappeared (MacArthur et al 1991), or became only marginally significant (Brown & Lumley 1998), after taking duration of second stage labour into account. Older maternal age, heavier infant birthweight and larger head circumference, as well as obesity and multiparity, have also been identified as risk factors for stress incontinence (MacArthur et al 1991, Viktrup et al 1992, Wilson et al 1996, Yarnell et al 1982). A combination of these various risk factors in the individual mother is likely to predispose to a particularly high risk of developing postpartum stress incontinence (MacArthur et al 1993).

Management

A combination of interventions for the management of stress incontinence may be appropriate, but further research is required to determine the optimum treatment for specific patient groups, including postpartum women. Behavioural techniques involve the use of pelvic floor exercises (PFE), either in isolation or combined with biofeedback therapy, or the use of weighted vaginal cones. Conservative treatment, involving PFE for diagnosed genuine stress incontinence and symptoms of stress incontinence, has been shown to be successful in observational and experimental general population studies when compared with other treatments or with no treatment (Bo et al 1999, Henalla et al 1988, Largo-Janssen et al 1991, Nygaard et al 1996). A recent systematic review, which included 11 general population trials, found good evidence of a benefit from PFE compared with no treatment, but the evidence was inconclusive with regard to other conservative therapies (Berghmans et al 1998).

There is little information, however, about the role and effectiveness of PFE in the postnatal period (Wilson et al 1987). Sleep & Grant (1987b) undertook a randomised controlled trial of the effects of an intensive PFE programme on the incidence of urinary incontinence at 3 months postpartum. The trial recruited 1800 women who had vaginal deliveries, all parities being included. Women were randomly allocated to either the intervention (intensive exercise programme) or the control group. Women in both groups received initial instruction in pelvic floor exercises from the hospital physiotherapist, which was standard practice. In addition, women in the intensive exercise group were instructed individually by a midwife coordinator, receiving an extra exercise session daily. At 3 months postpartum the prevalence of urinary incontinence was similar in both groups.

A recent multi-centre randomised controlled trial tested the effects of PFE and bladder training in the management of women who had postnatal incontinence at 3 months postpartum (Glazener et al 2001). Women (n = 747) were randomly allocated, after stratifying for mode of delivery, frequency of symptoms and parity (para $\geq$ 4 versus para $\leq$ 3), to the control (standard postnatal advice) or the intervention group, who received intensive home based instructions on PFE and bladder retraining from a specially trained midwife or health visitor at 5, 7 and 9 months postpartum. Assessment of outcome at 12 months, of 524 women (279 intervention and 245 control), found that significantly fewer of the intervention (167, 60%) than the control (169, 69%) group were still symptomatic. Perceived severity and frequency of symptoms were also less in the intervention group women. The population of this trial differed from the one previously described (Sleep & Grant 1987b) in that it included only symptomatic women.

Several small observational studies in general female populations have found PFE to be more successful in women with mild stress incontinence than in those with more severe forms (Elia & Bergman 1993, Mouritsen et al 1991, Wilson et al 1987); however the latter two studies included older women (50 years and above) and more information is required to assess the effect of PFE among younger women. It is likely that PFE are more likely to be effective if they are performed correctly, and adequate advice and training are necessary to do this (Bo et al 1988, Bump et al 1991, Morkved & Bo 1996, Wilson et al 1987).

URINARY TRACT INFECTION (UTI)
Definition

The urinary tract is considered to be infected if the bacterial count from two successive 'clean catch' urine samples or a single catheter sample exceeds 10^5/ml (Robertson & Hebert 1994). Urinary tract infections (UTI) are commonly reported during pregnancy, in some cases triggered by the presence of asymptomatic bacteriuria (ASB). A recent review reported that among the 2–10% of women who have ASB antenatally, about 40% subsequently develop symptoms of acute UTI (Cardozo & Gleeson 1997). Obstetric teaching is that UTIs may ascend from the urethra (urethritis) to the bladder (cystitis) or to the kidney (pyelonephritis) (Robertson & Herbert 1994). The presenting symptoms will, to some extent, determine the site of the infection. For example, if presenting symptoms include suprapubic discomfort and urinary frequency but the patient is afebrile, cystitis would be the most likely diagnosis. Flank pain, nausea or vomiting, pyrexia and renal angle tenderness would suggest upper urinary tract involvement (Donohoe 1995). Frank haematuria is occasionally seen, but can be indicative of other pathology.

Treatment of UTI is often instituted on clinical symptoms as urine culture takes several days. In symptomatic populations, estimates of the sensitivity of dipstick tests for nitrites (produced by reduction of nitrate in urine by infecting organisms) are between 45% and 83% (Barker et al 1989, Evans et al 1991, Lowe 1985, Mills et al 1992).

Frequency of occurrence and risk factors

Limited information on the incidence and prevalence of postpartum UTI suggests that around 2–4% of women develop this after childbirth (Craigo & Kapermick 1994). Stray-Pederson et al (1990), in a study of 6803 puerperal patients comprising all women delivering during a 2 year period in one Norwegian maternity unit, found an incidence of 'true' bacteriuria of 3.7% (assessed first from voided MSU, followed by suprapubic aspiration sample), only 21% of whom complained of dysuria. Risk factors of UTI were found to be a history of UTI, caesarean and instrumental delivery, epidural anaesthesia and bladder catheterisation, although analyses did not take account of inter-relationships between factors. Schwartz et al (1999) carried out a retrospective case control study of women who delivered in one American state between 1987 and 1993 to investigate postpartum risk factors of UTI. Cases were those diagnosed with a UTI as designated by the International Classification of Diseases – 10 and recorded on the hospital discharge information (n = 931), and these were matched with two randomly selected controls (n = 1862) who had no diagnosis of UTI on discharge. An increased risk for postpartum UTI, after undertaking multivariate analysis to control for confounders, was found for caesarean delivery, induction of labour, pre-eclampsia or eclampsia, placental abruption, renal disease, unmarried status and Black or Hispanic race.

Some information on UTI has been obtained from studies of post-caesarean section infections, although most were hospital based with only short term follow-up. Following this mode of delivery, infection rates of 11–35% have been reported (Buchholz et al 1994, Leigh et al 1990, Parrott et al 1989). In one small prospective study of 124 women delivered by caesarean section, 18 (14%) developed a UTI (Parrott et al 1989). Leigh et al (1990) studied postoperative infections of the genitourinary tract in women who had a caesarean delivery in 1985 and 1987 at one UK maternity unit, where catheterisation was routine, although techniques varied in the two periods studied. In 1985, 62 (34%) of 183 women developed post-catheterisation bacteriuria within 2 days, as did 49 (25%) of the 192 women who had sections in 1987. The authors considered that post-catheterisation bacteriuria was reduced by improved catheterisation techniques. Buchholz et al (1994), in a retrospective case note analysis of 1438 sections in one unit in Switzerland between 1985 and 1990, found that significant bacteriuria had been recorded in 11.6% of the women (the number who developed symptomatic UTI was not presented). In this unit postoperative catheterisation was routine, with a mean duration of 2.3 days. In both of the last two studies it was stated that prophylactic antibiotics were not administered to the women undergoing caesarean section, and it is likely that this could have had an effect on the numbers who developed postoperative UTI and other infectious morbidities (refer to section on management below).

Management

A large number of different antibiotic regimens are used to treat UTI in women, but there is debate as to the relative effectiveness of short term treatment classed as single dose, treatment for 3 days or treatment for 5 days (or longer) in relation to costs, patient compliance and adverse reactions (Bandolier 1995). In the Norwegian study described earlier (Stray-Pederson et al 1990), the 251 cases of UTI were randomly allocated to different treatments. Of the 153 with amoxicillin-susceptible bacteria, 1, 3 and 10 days duration treatment of amoxicillin were given (how these were allocated is not clear), showing cure rates of 84%, 94% and 98%. The cure rate among 46 women who had amoxicillin-resistant bacteriuria, and who received cefalexin or nitrofurantoin for 7 days, was 91%. 52 women received no treatment (again unclear how these were selected), 27% of whom still had persistent bacteriuria when tested 10 weeks later. These authors concluded that for confirmed postpartum bladder bacteriuria, 3 days of therapy appears to be sufficient.

Ragnar Norrby (1990) carried out a systematic review of trials that compared different duration and types of treatment for UTIs among the general female population; 28 trials were included involving over 3000 women. The review found that irrespective of which antibiotic was used, single dose treatment of cystitis was less effective than 3 day or 5 day (or longer) treatments. Differences between 3 day and 5 day treatments, however, varied according to which types of antibiotic were used. With trimethoprim/sulfonamide combinations adverse reactions increased markedly when treatment was given for more than 3 days, so the authors recommended that these should not be continued for longer than 3 days.

Treatment of UTI will vary according to whether the infection is confined to the lower or upper urinary tract or if there are any complicating factors, such as renal disease. A recent Cochrane systematic review concluded that prophylactic antibiotics for women who deliver by caesarean section will reduce the risk of postpartum UTI, as well as other infectious morbidities (Smaill & Hofmeyr 2000).

The use of cranberry juice in the management of UTI has been suggested as being beneficial because certain properties in the berries are thought to reduce bacteria. However, one systematic review to examine the use of cranberries in the prevention of UTI and another to examine treatment (Jepson et al 1999a, 1999b) concluded that, due to the small number of poor quality trials, there is no evidence of any effect of cranberry juice on UTI.

If there is pain associated with a UTI, it is common practice to advise analgesia. Paracetamol may be tried in the first instance but for further guidance see 'Simple Pain Relief' in Guideline No.3.

DETRUSOR INSTABILITY

Detrusor instability is the second most common cause of urinary incontinence in women and diagnosis is usually made following urodynamic investigations. Unstable contractions which cannot be suppressed by the patient increase the pressure in the bladder and may result in urge incontinence, defined as the involuntary loss of urine associated with a strong desire to void (Abrams et al 1990), frequency and nocturia (Kelleher et al 1997). The incidence of detrusor instability increases with age (Cardozo & Khullar 1995) and is higher among women than men (Couillard & Webster 1995).

No studies have been identified that have examined detrusor instability among postnatal women. It is considered to be more common during pregnancy but most cases are likely to resolve in the puerperium (Cardozo & Gleeson 1997). Some studies have documented the prevalence of specific related symptoms, such as urge incontinence, which may have been associated with a diagnosis of detrusor instability had this been investigated. For example Wilson et al (1996), in the observational study of postnatal incontinence in New Zealand referred to earlier, found that 10.4% of the women in the sample reported symptoms of urge incontinence at 3 months postpartum. Cutner (1995) questioned a sample of 119 women during pregnancy and after delivery and found a postpartum prevalence of 6% of urge incontinence and 19% of urgency. Symptom prevalences had been higher during pregnancy.

Assassa et al (2000), in a general population community survey of over 6000 women with a median age of 58 years, found urge incontinence (OR 1.29) and nocturia (OR 1.33) at the time of questioning to be significantly more likely in women who had ever delivered a baby over 4 kg.

URINARY RETENTION AND VOIDING DIFFICULTIES

Postpartum urinary retention is known to occur but the exact incidence is difficult to ascertain since retention is variably defined. Yip et al (1997) found that among 691 vaginal deliveries, 14.6% had retention on day 1, defined as a residual urinary volume of 150 ml or more. Lee et al (1999) defined postpartum urinary retention as a residual volume exceeding 200 ml on day 2, and found this in 14.1% of 256 vaginal births. Saultz et al (1991), in a literature review, reported a range of incidence of between 1.7% and 17.9%. Retention can be asymptomatic. In addition to having epidural analgesia (see below), risk factors for retention have been found to be caesarean section, instrumental delivery and prolonged labour (Lee et al 1999, Saultz et al 1991, Yip et al 1997).

Epidural analgesia can impede the usual sensory impulses in the bladder, and several studies have found this to be a risk factor for urinary retention (Ramsay & Torbet 1993, Weil et al 1983). Weil et al (1983) undertook a urodynamic study of 27 primiparous women to ascertain the effect of epidurals on lower urinary tract function. They found that hypotonic bladders were more common among women delivered vaginally with epidural analgesia. The authors noted that the group was too small to enable definite conclusions but suggested that patients with epidural analgesia should be monitored for bladder distension. Khullar & Cardozo (1993), in a study of bladder sensation after epidural analgesia, found that it took up to 8 hours for the bladder to regain sensation, and within this time more than 1 litre of urine could be produced, which could subsequently damage detrusor function.

Cardozo & Gleeson (1997) have suggested that, in order for overdistension after epidural to be prevented, an indwelling urethral catheter should be inserted at the time of the epidural block and left in situ for 12 hours after the last top-up. Whether mobile epidurals, using lower concentrations of anaesthetic agents, have a different effect is not known. More information on the effects of epidural analgesia on the bladder, and on the most effective management of urinary retention, is required.

URINARY FISTULAE

Urinary fistulae are classified according to the organs between which they are established (uterovaginal, vesicovaginal, urethrovaginal or complex), and are usually a consequence of obstetric trauma. They are a major problem in developing countries where there is limited medical care (Elkins 1994) and known to be rare in developed countries, although prevalence rates for the UK are not available. Vesicovaginal fistulae are the most common, developing between the bladder and vagina as a result of devitalisation of tissue at the bladder base, caused either by direct pressure from the fetal head on the symphysis pubis or by trauma during a difficult instrumental delivery. One midwifery textbook describes that sloughing of the devitalised area can take between 8 and 12 days, when the mother may develop incontinence of urine (Abbott 1997). Incontinence of urine is continuous and the fistula is usually visible on speculum examination (Cardozo 1991).

Vesicovaginal fistulae can be treated conservatively with bladder drainage and antibiotics, during which time a few will heal spontaneously (Cardozo 1991); however it is not known how long this would take. Vaginal or abdominal repair is generally performed 2–3 months after the initial injury (Cardozo 1991). Reports of surgical management of vesicovaginal fistulae usually comprise case series from hospitals in developing countries (Waaldijk 1994). Although rare in the developed world, any woman who has had a traumatic labour and/or delivery who reports a continuous leakage of urine should be immediately referred to the GP and a diagnosis of fistula excluded.

SUMMARY OF THE EVIDENCE USED IN THIS GUIDELINE

- Evidence from large well conducted observational studies shows that stress incontinence after childbirth is widespread and persistent and may have an effect on women's lifestyles.
- Evidence from randomised controlled trials, including general population samples and one of symptomatic postpartum women, suggests a benefit from performing pelvic floor exercises (PFE); however further evidence is required to confirm effects in the postnatal period.
- A systematic review of prophylactic antibiotics following caesarean sections concluded that postoperative infectious morbidity, including infection of the lower urinary tract, will be reduced.
- A general female population based systematic review has shown that single short treatment for cystitis is less effective than longer durations.
- Overdistention of the bladder has been shown in observational studies to be more likely to occur after epidural analgesia. More evidence on this is required.

WHAT TO DO

INITIAL ASSESSMENT

- Ask about history of present problem
  - What is the main complaint or symptom and its duration?
- Ask about the following symptoms
  - Frequency (expert opinion suggests this is the need to pass urine more than seven times a day or more often than every 2 hours)
  - Incontinence (stress and urge)
  - Retention/voiding difficulties (such as feeling of incomplete emptying of the bladder; poor stream; straining to void; dysuria; inability to void; awareness of full bladder)
  - Haematuria (blood in urine).
- Dipstix fresh urine sample: if positive for nitrites treat as UTI; if negative send MSU to exclude UTI.
- Ask if the bladder problem interferes with routine activities, or if she finds it troublesome in any other way.
- Does the woman need to wear protective pads?

CONDITIONS WHICH REQUIRE IMMEDIATE REFERRAL TO GP

- Retention of urine (expert opinion suggests post-void residual volume >100 ml).
- Heavily blood stained urine.
- Frank incontinence.
- Urine leaking from vagina.

STRESS INCONTINENCE

- Exclude/detect possible underlying causes: UTI, urinary retention.
- If there is no evidence of a UTI it is common practice to advise normal fluid intake (not more than 2 litres per day).
- Give instructions on how to do pelvic floor exercises, to perform daily. (See pages 99,102 for instructions.)
- If appropriate refer to the district continence advisor, e.g. if the woman requires protective pads, or finds the condition interferes with routine tasks. (This will be according to local policy—the hospital physiotherapist will be able to advise you on how best to contact him/her if this service is available.)
- Reassess symptoms at subsequent visits and if condition becomes worse refer to district continence advisor after excluding possible underlying causes.
- If the condition has not improved by the time of final postnatal check with GP advise that she tells the GP about this. (If final postnatal check is undertaken by the midwife, referral to the GP should be made.)

Confirmed UTI (i.e. dipstix shows positive nitrites or MSU shows positive culture)

- Refer to GP for antibiotics.
- Although there is no evidence base, it is common practice to advise increased fluid intake (i.e. more than 2 litres per day).
- If analgesia is required give paracetamol (refer to 'Simple Pain Relief' in Guideline 3).

Urinary retention and voiding difficulties

- Define specific problem. If retention suspected, expert opinion suggests that post-micturition residual volume via in/out catheter should be measured: if volume >100 ml *refer immediately to GP.*
- It is common practice to suggest warm bath or shower might assist micturition.
- If condition causes a problem irrespective of post-micturition residual volume, refer to GP.
- Reassess at subsequent visits; if condition worsens or does not resolve refer to GP.

How to perform PFE

- Ask the woman what information she has received about PFE and make sure she has any leaflets available from the maternity unit physiotherapy department. Work through the leaflets with her. The following regime is suggested by the Association of Chartered Physiotherapists in Women's Health.
- Tell the mother to get into a comfortable position (any position will do) and imagine that you are trying to stop yourself from passing wind and at the same time trying to stop your flow of urine. The feeling is one of 'squeeze and lift', closing and drawing-up the back and front passages. This is called a **pelvic floor contraction.**
- **Remember** – you should start gently and stop if it hurts. Don't pull in your stomach excessively, squeeze your legs together, tighten your buttocks or hold your breath.
- This programme is designed to build up the endurance of the pelvic floor muscles, so that they will be able to work harder and longer. Firstly, though, you'll need to determine your 'starting block'.
- Tighten your pelvic floor muscles as previously described and hold for as many seconds as you can (maximum of 10 seconds).
- Release the contraction and rest for 4 seconds. Then repeat the 'tighten, hold and release' movement as many times as you can (up to a maximum of 10).
- For example, if you can hold the contraction for 2 seconds and repeat 4 times, this is your 'starting block'.
- Now perform the basic pelvic floor exercise – but squeeze and lift more firmly, then let go. This is called a **quick contraction** and will help your muscles react quickly when you laught, cough, sneeze, exercise or lift.
- Aim to increase the number of quick contractions, up to a maximum of 10.

(Taken from: *Fit for motherhood*, a leaflet produced by the Association of Chartered Physiotherapists in Women's Health)

SUMMARY GUIDELINE

URINARY PROBLEMS

INITIAL ASSESSMENT

- Obtain history of present problem
- Ask about the following symptoms:
  - Frequency
  - Incontinence (stress and urge)
  - Voiding difficulties/retention
  - Haematuria
- Dipstix fresh urine sample; if positive nitrites treat as UTI, if negative send MSU
- Does the problem interfere with routine activities?
- Does the woman need to wear protective pads?

IMMEDIATE REFERRAL TO GP IS REQUIRED IF:

- Retention of urine (expert opinion suggests post-void residual vol >100 ml)
- Heavily blood stained urine
- Frank incontinence
- Urine leakage from vagina

WHAT TO DO

STRESS INCONTINENCE

- Exclude possible underlying causes such as UTI, retention of urine
- If no evidence of UTI, advise *normal* fluid intake (no more than 2 litres per day)
- Give instructions on pelvic floor exercises to perform daily
- If appropriate, refer to the district continence advisor, e.g. if the woman continues to require protective pads, or finds the condition interferes with routine tasks
- Reassess symptoms at subsequent visits. If condition becomes worse refer to district continence advisor after excluding underlying causes
- If not improved by the final postnatal check, refer to GP

CONFIRMED UTI

- Refer to GP for antibiotics
- Although there is no evidence base, advise increased fluid intake (i.e. at least 2 litres per day)
- If required give analgesia as local prescribing policy

URINARY RETENTION AND VOIDING DIFFICULTIES

- Define specific problem. If retention suspected measure post-micturition residual volume via in/out catheter: if volume >100 ml refer immediately to GP
- Suggest warm bath or shower might assist micturition
- Reassess at subsequent visits; if condition worsens or unresolved by the final postnatal check, refer to GP

HOW TO PERFORM PELVIC FLOOR EXERCISES

Ask woman what information she has received about PFE, provide leaflets if necessary and work through with her.

To do your pelvic floor exercises, first get into a comfortable position (any position will do) and follow these instructions.

Imagine that you are trying to stop yourself from passing wind and at the same time trying to stop your flow of urine. The feeling is one of 'squeeze and lift', closing and drawing-up the back and front passages. This is called a **pelvic floor contraction**.

Remember—*you should start gently and stop if it hurts. Don't pull in your stomach excessively, squeeze your legs together, tighten your buttocks or hold your breath.*

This programme is designed to build up the endurance of the pelvic floor muscles, so that they will be able to work harder and longer. Firstly, though, you'll need to determine your 'starting block'.

Tighten your pelvic floor muscles as previously described and hold for as many seconds as you can (maximum of 10 seconds).

Release the contraction and rest for 4 seconds. Then repeat the 'tighten, hold and release' movement as many times as you can (up to a maximum of 10).

For example, if you can hold the contraction for 2 seconds and repeat four times, this is your 'starting block'.

Now perform the basic pelvic floor exercise—but squeeze and lift more firmly, then let go. This is called a **quick contraction** *and will help your muscles react quickly when you laugh, cough, sneeze, exercise or lift.*

Aim to increase the number of quick contractions, up to a maximum of 10.

(Taken from: *FIT for motherhood*, a leaflet produced by the Association of Chartered Physiotherapists in Women's Health)

REFERENCES

Abbott H 1997 Complications of the puerperium. In: Sweet B (ed) Mayes midwifery. A textbook for midwives, 12th edn. Baillière Tindall, London, pp 719–729

Abrams P, Blaivas J G, Stanton S L et al 1990 The standardisation of terminology of the lower urinary tract function. Br J Obstet Gynaecol 97 (suppl 6): 1–16

Allen R E, Hosker G L, Smith A R B 1990 Pelvic floor damage and childbirth: a neurophysiological study. Br J Obstet Gynaecol 97: 770–779

Assassa L P, Dallosso S, Perry C et al, and the Leicestershire MRC Incontinence Study Team 2000 The association between obstetric factors and incontinence: a community survey. Br J Obstet Gynaecol 107: 822

Bandolier (newsletter) 1995 Drug watch: antimicrobial treatment of cystitis. Bandolier 13: 3

Barker B A, Ratcliffe G, Turner G C 1989 Urine screening for leucocytes and bacteriuria by dipstick and reflectance spectrophotometry. Med Lab Sciences 46: 97–100

Berghmans L C, Hendriks H J, Bo K et al 1998 Conservative treatment of stress urinary incontinence in women: a systematic review of randomised clinical trials. Br J Urol 82: 181–191

Bick D E, MacArthur C 1995 The extent, severity and effect of health problems after childbirth. Br J Midwif 3: 27–31

Bo K et al 1988 Knowledge about and the ability to correct pelvic floor muscle exercises in women with urinary stress incontinence. Neurourol Urodyn 7: 261

Bo K, Talseth T, Holme I 1999 Single blind, randomised controlled trial of pelvic floor exercises, electrical stimulation, vaginal cones, and no treatment in management of genuine stress incontinence in women. BMJ 318: 487–493

Brown S, Lumley J 1998 Maternal health after childbirth: results of an Australian population based survey. Br J Obstet Gynaecol 105: 156–161

Buchholz N-P, Daly-Grandeau E, Huber-Buchholz M-M 1994 Urological complications associated with caesarean section. Eur J Obstet Gynecol Reprod Biol 56: 161–163

Bump R C, Hurt W G, Fantl J A, Wyman J F 1991 Assessment of Kegel pelvic muscle exercise performance after brief verbal instruction. Am J Obstet Gynecol 165(2): 322–329

Burgio K L, Matthews K A, Engell B T 1991 Prevalence, incidence and correlates of urinary incontinence in healthy, middle-aged women. J Urol 146: 1255–1259

Cardozo L 1991 Urinary incontinence in women: have we anything new to offer? BMJ 303: 1453–1457

Cardozo L, Gleeson C 1997 Pregnancy, childbirth and continence. Br J Midwif 5(5): 277–281

Cardozo K, Khullar V 1995 Detrusor instability—drugs and behavioural therapies. In: Smith A R B (ed) Urogynaecology. The investigation and management of urinary incontinence in women. RCOG Press, London

Couillard D R, Webster G D 1995 Detrusor instability. Urol Clin N Am 22(3): 593–612

Craigo S D, Kapermick P S 1994 Postpartum haemorrhage and the abnormal puerperium. In: DeCherney A H, Pernoll M L (eds) Current obstetric and gynaecological diagnosis and treatment, 8th edn. Prentice Hall International, London

Cutner A 1995 The bladder in pregnancy and the puerperium. In: Smith A R B (ed) Urogynaecology. The investigation and management of urinary incontinence in women. RCOG Press, London

Dimpfl T, Hesse U, Schussler B 1992 Incidence and cause of postpartum urinary stress incontinence. Eur J Obstet Gynecol Reprod Biol 43: 29–33

Donohoe J 1995 Urinary tract infection in women (editorial). Ir Med J 88(5): 142–143

Elia G A, Bergman A 1993 Pelvic muscle exercises: when do they work? Obstet Gynecol 81(2): 283–286

Elkins T E 1994 Surgery for the obstetric vesicovaginal fistula: a review of 100 operations in 82 patients. Am J Obstet Gynecol 170(4): 1108–1120

Evans P J, Leaker B R, McNabb W R, Lewis R R 1991 Accuracy of reagent strip testing for urinary tract infection. J Roy Soc Med 84: 598–599

Glazener C M A, Herbison G P, Wilson P D, MacArthur C, Lang G D, Gee H, Grant H M Conservative management of persistent postnatal urinary and faecal incontinence: a randomised controlled trial. BMJ In press

Henalla S M, Kirwan P, Castleden C M et al 1988 The effect of pelvic floor exercises in the treatment of genuine urinary stress incontinence in women at two hospitals. Br J Obstet Gynaecol 95: 602–606

Holst K Y, Wilson P D 1988 The prevalence of female urinary incontinence and reasons for not seeking treatment. N Z Med J 101: 756–758

Jepson R G, Mihaljevic L, Craig J 1999a Cranberries for preventing urinary tract infections. Cochrane Review 4. The Cochrane Library, Oxford

Jepson R G, Mihaljevic L, Craig J 1999b Cranberries for treating urinary tract infections. Cochrane Review 4. The Cochrane Library, Oxford

Jolleys J V 1988 Reported prevalence of urinary incontinence in women in a general practice. BMJ 296: 1300–1302

Kelleher C J, Cardozo L D, Khullar V et al 1997 A medium term analysis of the subjective efficacy of treatment for women with detrusor instability and low bladder compliance. Br J Obstet Gynaecol 104: 988–993

Khullar V, Cardozo L D 1993 Bladder sensation after epidural analgesia. Neurourol Urodyn 12: 424–425

Largo-Janssen T L M, Debruyne F M J, Smits A J A et al 1991 Controlled trial of pelvic floor exercises in the treatment of urinary stress incontinence in general practice. Br J Gen Pract 41: 445–449

Lee S N S, Lee C P, Tang O S F et al 1999 Postpartum urinary retention. Int J Gynaecol Obstet 66: 287–288

Leigh D A, Emmanuel F X S, Sedgwick J et al 1990 Post-operative urinary tract infection and wound infection in women undergoing Caesarean section: a comparison of two study periods in 1985 and 1987. J Hosp Infect 15: 107–116

Lowe P A 1985 Chemical screening and prediction of bacteriuria – a new approach. Med Lab Sciences 42: 23–28

MacArthur C, Lewis M, Knox E G 1991 Health after childbirth. HMSO, London

MacArthur C, Lewis M, Bick D E 1993 Stress incontinence after childbirth. Br J Midwif 1(5): 207–215

Mason L, Glenn S, Walton I et al 1999 The experience of stress incontinence after childbirth. Birth 26(3): 164–171

Meyer S, Schreyer A, DeGrandi P et al 1998 The effects of birth on urinary continence: mechanisms and other pelvic-floor characteristics. Obstet Gynecol 92: 613–618

Mills S J, Ford M, Gould K, Burton S, Neal D E 1992 Screening for bacteriuria in urological patients using reagent strips. Br J Urology 70: 314–317

Morkved S, Bo K 1996 The effect of post-natal exercises to strengthen the pelvic floor muscles. Acta Obstet Gynecol Scand 75: 382–385

Mouritsen L, Frimodt-Moller C, Møller M 1991 Long-term effect of pelvic floor exercises on female urinary incontinence. Br J Urol 68: 32–37

Nygaard I E, Kreder K J, Lepic M M et al 1996 Efficacy of pelvic floor muscle exercises in women with stress, urge, and mixed urinary incontinence. Am J Obstet Gynecol 174(1): 120–125

O'Brien J, Austin M, Sethi P et al 1991 Urinary incontinence: prevalence, need for treatment, and effectiveness of intervention by nurse. BMJ 303: 1308–1312

Parrott T, Evans A J, Lowes A et al 1989 Infection following caesarean section. J Hosp Infect 13: 349–354

Ragnar Norrby S 1990 Short-term treatment of uncomplicated lower urinary tract infections in women. Rev Infect Dis 12(3): 458–467

Ramsay I N, Torbet T E 1993 Incidence of abnormal voiding parameters in the immediate postpartum period. Neurourol Urodyn 12(2): 179–183

Robertson J R, Hebert D B 1994 Gynecologic urology. In: DeCherney A H, Pernoll M L (eds) Current obstetric and gynaecological diagnosis and treatment, 8th edn. Prentice Hall International, London, ch 42, pp 831–845

Saultz J W, Toffler W L, Shackles J Y 1991 Postpartum urinary retention. J Am Board Fam Pract 4(5): 341–344

Saurel-Cubizolles M-J, Romito P, Lelong N et al 2000 Women's health after childbirth: a longitudinal study in France and Italy. Br J Obstet Gynaecol 107: 1202–1209

Schwartz M A, Wang C C, Eckert L O et al 1999 Risk factors for urinary tract infection in the postpartum period. Am J Obstet Gynecol 181(3): 547–553

Sleep J, Grant A 1987a West Berkshire perineal management trial: three year follow-up. BMJ 295: 749–751

Sleep J, Grant A 1987b Pelvic floor exercises in postnatal care—the report of a randomised controlled trial to compare an intensive exercise regimen with the programme in current use. Midwifery 3: 158–164

Sleep J, Grant A, Garcia J et al 1984 West Berkshire perineal management trial. BMJ 289: 587–590

Smaill F, Hofmeyr G J 2000 Antibiotic prophylaxis for Caesarean section. Cochrane Review 3. The Cochrane Library, Oxford

Snooks S J, Setchell M, Swash M et al 1984 Injury to the innervation of pelvic floor sphincter musculature in childbirth. Lancet II: 546–550

Snooks S J, Swash M, Henry M M et al 1986 Risk factors in childbirth causing damage to the pelvic floor innervation. Int J Colorectal Dis 1: 20–24

Stray-Pederson B, Blakstad M, Bergan T 1990 Bacteriuria in the puerperium: risk factors, screening procedures, and treatment programs. Am J Obstet Gynecol 162(3): 792–797

Thomas T M, Plymat K R, Blannin J et al 1980 Prevalence of urinary incontinence. BMJ 281: 1243–1245

Viktrup L, Lose G, Rolff M et al 1992 The symptoms of stress incontinence caused by pregnancy or delivery in primiparas. Obstet Gynecol 79(6): 945–949

Waaldijk K 1994 The immediate surgical-management of fresh obstetric fistulas with catheter and/or early closure. Int J Gynecol Obstet 45(1): 11–16

Weil A, Reyes H, Rottenberg R D et al 1983 Effect of lumbar epidural analgesia on lower urinary tract function in the immediate postpartum period. Br J Obstet Gynaecol 90: 428–432

Wilson P D, Samarrai T, Deakin M et al 1987 An objective assessment of physiotherapy for female genuine stress incontinence. Br J Obstet Gynaecol 94: 575–582

Wilson P D, Herbison R M, Herbison G P 1996 Obstetric practice and the prevalence of urinary incontinence three months after delivery. Br J Obstet Gynaecol 103: 154–161

Yarnell J W G, Voyle G J, Richards C J et al 1981 The prevalence and severity of urinary incontinence in women. J Epidemiol Community Health 35: 71–74

Yarnell J W G, Voyle G J, Sweetnam P M et al 1982 Factors associated with urinary incontinence in women. J Epidemiol Community Health 36: 58–63

Yip S-K, Brieger G, Hin L-Y 1997 Urinary retention in the post-partum period. The relationship between obstetric factors and the post-partum post-void residual bladder volume. Acta Obstet Gynecol Scand 76: 667–672

6

Bowel problems

INTRODUCTION

There are various bowel problems that women can experience following childbirth. Constipation and haemorrhoids have long been known as common postpartum symptoms, and recent studies have shown that women may also experience anal fissure (Corby et al 1997) or fecal incontinence in the postpartum period. Third degree tear is included in this guideline because of the high risk of subsequent bowel control problems.

CONSTIPATION

Definition

Constipation is defined as difficulty evacuating the bowel and can be associated with various factors, including an inadequate intake of dietary fibre and physical or psychological illness. It is a common symptom during the second and third trimester of pregnancy, arising from relaxation of the smooth muscle of the intestine as a result of circulating progesterone (Shepherd 1997). During the postpartum period women may experience constipation following lack of dietary intake during labour or because of pain from perineal trauma.

Frequency of occurrence and risk factors

Although it is generally 'well known' that constipation can occur after childbirth, there is little documentary evidence of its prevalence or risk factors. Garcia & Marchant (1993), as part of an in depth descriptive survey of postnatal care, sent 100 women a postal questionnaire at 8 weeks postpartum to ask about health problems: 90 women responded, 20 (22%) of whom had experienced constipation since their delivery, although onset and duration were not given. In a prospective observational study in Scotland, a representative sample of over 1200 women were surveyed whilst still in hospital, at 8 weeks and at 12–18 months, when half the sample was followed up to ask about symptoms after 8 weeks: 19%, 20% and 7% respectively reported constipation at these various times (Glazener et al 1995). In a longitudinal survey by Saurel-Cubizolles et al (2000), 13% of the Italian women and 14% of the French reported constipation at 5 months. At 12 months these proportions were 17% and 26% respectively.

At all survey periods in the study by Glazener et al (1995), univariate analysis showed that constipation was significantly more common among women following instrumental deliveries, compared with spontaneous vaginal deliveries or caesarean sections. The proportions reporting constipation were, respectively, 31%, 17% and 20% in hospital; 31%, 18% and 17% between then and 8 weeks, and 14%, 6% and 5% after this. Constipation whilst still in hospital was found to be more common among primiparae (23%) than multiparae (16%), but after this the parity difference was non-significant (Glazener et al 1995). Since primiparae have much higher rates of instrumental deliveries than multiparae, the parity association may not be an independent one. French women who reported constipation at 12 months in the survey by Saurel-Cubizolles et al (2000) were more likely to be in employment, but there was no similar difference among the Italian women.

Management

There is limited research into the most effective treatment of constipation among either obstetric or non-obstetric populations and most conservative management of postpartum constipation is based on current clinical practice.

Jewell & Young (2000), in a Cochrane systematic review of interventions for the treatment of constipation during pregnancy, could find only one trial on this. These findings, based on 40 women, showed that bran and wheat supplements were effective in increasing the frequency of defecation (OR 0.18, 95% CI 0.05–0.67) and unlikely to have side effects for the mother or fetus. In an early randomised controlled trial in South Africa, comparing the use of the laxative senna (n = 224) with placebo (n = 247) for immediate postpartum constipation, senna was shown to be effective in producing spontaneous bowel action, but 12% of cases compared with 3% of controls experienced abdominal cramps, although most were described as mild (Shelton 1980).

Tramonte et al (1997) undertook a systematic review of general population trials (peripartum trials excluded) to evaluate whether laxatives and fibre therapy, for a minimum of 1 week, improved symptoms in adults who had experienced constipation for at least 2 weeks. 36 trials were included, with a total of 1815 subjects, and a range of different laxative and fibre treatments. The reviewers concluded that both fibre and laxatives modestly improved bowel movement frequency but there was insufficient evidence to determine whether fibre was superior to laxative treatment or whether one class of laxative was better than another. They suggested that laxatives should only be given when simple treatments, fibre and dietary interventions, have failed.

As discussed later, constipation in the postnatal period has been shown to be associated with the development of acute anal fissure (Corby et al 1997).

HAEMORRHOIDS

Definition

Haemorrhoids result from swollen veins around the anus, which in severe cases can prolapse. Haemorrhoids can be graded according to the degree of prolapse; first degree haemorrhoids are visible but do not prolapse; second degree haemorrhoids prolapse with defecation but return spontaneously; third degree haemorrhoids prolapse and require manual replacement; and fourth degree haemorrhoids remain prolapsed outside of the anal canal (Pfenninger 1997). During pregnancy, haemorrhoids may occur as a result of the action of progesterone on the bowel which increases varicosity; and during the postnatal period possibly as a consequence of pushing in the second stage of labour.

Frequency of occurrence and risk factors

Like constipation, haemorrhoids are a 'well known' consequence of childbirth. Midwifery and obstetric textbooks have generally noted that haemorrhoids can cause a great deal of pain for a few days after delivery, but then resolve, although they may worsen with subsequent pregnancies, and can eventually become permanent (Hibbard 1988). More recently, however, information from observational studies of health problems after childbirth have found that haemorrhoids, whether of pregnancy or postpartum onset, do not always resolve quickly. MacArthur et al (1991), in an observational study, found that among 11 701 women, 8% reported haemorrhoids of more than 6 weeks duration starting for the first time within 3 months of birth, and an additional 10% reported these as ongoing or recurrent symptoms. Two thirds of the women reporting haemorrhoids still had them at the time of questioning, 1–9 years after delivery. Multivariate analysis showed that new symptoms were independently associated with a forceps delivery, a longer second stage of labour and with the vaginal delivery of a heavier baby. They were less likely after caesarean section and if delivered by section, heavier birthweight had no effect. All these associations are compatible with a longer or more expulsive period of pushing.

Glazener et al (1995), in the study referred to earlier, found that 17% of women reported haemorrhoids (new and recurrent) when questioned in hospital, 22% between then and 8 weeks and 15% after this. As in the study by MacArthur et al (1991), women who had an instrumental delivery were significantly more likely to report haemorrhoids than those who had a spontaneous vaginal delivery, and those delivered by caesarean section were significantly less likely: 27%, 17% and 6% respectively whilst in hospital; and 31%, 23% and 14% between then and 8 weeks. When questioned at 12–18 months, however, no difference was found in the proportion who had experienced haemorrhoids after 8 weeks in the SVD (13%) compared with the caesarean section group (11%), but significantly more women still experienced haemorrhoids in the instrumental delivery group (30%). The effects of other factors, such as duration of second stage labour or birthweight, were not reported. Brown & Lumley (1998), in an Australian survey at 6–7 months postpartum, also found haemorrhoids to be significantly associated with mode of delivery, occurring after 36% of instrumental deliveries, 25% of spontaneous vaginal deliveries, 17% of elective and 11% of emergency sections. In the survey by Saurel-Cubizolles et al (2000) there was a high prevalence of haemorrhoids among French and Italian women at 5 months (16% and 16% in both cases), and these proportions increased at 12 months to 21% among Italian women and 26% among the French. The authors suggest various reasons for the 12 months increase in symptoms, including a change in women's perception of their health, which by then may feel more bothersome, as well as perhaps the effect of the increasing demands of the baby.

Management

Treatment options available for haemorrhoids are varied and generally depend on severity, with scalpel surgery now reserved only for advanced fourth degree cases (Pfenninger 1997). Relief of mild symptoms may be provided by the topical application of creams, and dietary advice to ensure avoidance of constipation is also usually given, although there is no trial evidence of the effectiveness of this treatment in a postpartum population. As with constipation, the conservative management of less severe childbirth related haemorrhoids is based on current clinical practice.

If haemorrhoids are severe and further treatment is required there are now numerous options, including rubber band ligation, cryothermy, injection sclerotherapy, infrared coagulation and diathermy as well as operative haemorrhoidectomy (MacRae & McLeod 1995, Pfenninger 1997). One meta-analysis, of 18 randomised controlled trials comparing the effectiveness of different treatments in the general population, concluded that rubber band ligation should be recommended as first line treatment for grade 1–3 haemorrhoids (MacRae & McLeod 1995). This procedure can be very painful however (Hardwick & Durdey 1994), and local anaesthetic injection to reduce postligation discomfort may only give very short benefit (Hooker et al 1999). Another review, including five trials of rubber band ligation, injection sclerotherapy and infrared coagulation, concluded that although rubber band ligation demonstrated greater long term efficacy, infrared coagulation may be the preferred treatment because it was associated with fewer and less severe complications (Johanson & Rimm 1992). There have been no trials identified which have specifically evaluated treatments for severe haemorrhoids in the postpartum period.

ANAL FISSURE

Definition

Anal fissure is a split or tear in the skin of the anal canal, usually in the posterior midline (Brisinda et al 1999). It is characterised by pain on defecation, which is usually severe, rectal bleeding and spasm of the internal anal sphincter (Lund & Scholefield 1997).

Frequency of occurrence and risk factors

There are few studies of postpartum anal fissure, but a group in Dublin recently carried out a prospective investigation in a sample of 313 primiparous women (Corby et al 1997). The diagnosis of anal fissure was made by clinical history and examination at, or before, the 6 week postnatal check. A detailed bowel questionnaire and obstetric details were also recorded. A total of 29 cases of anal fissure were found, an incidence of 9%, although the authors note that without the detailed nature of the follow-up in their study, many of the women would have been diagnosed as having 'acute painful haemorrhoids' (Corby et al 1997). Type of delivery, perineal trauma (tear, episiotomy, sutures) were not found to differ between the fissure and no fissure groups, nor was the use of epidural analgesia. 209 of the women in this study had anal manometry 6 weeks before and after delivery (the remainder only had this antenatally), which showed that mean maximum resting and squeeze anal canal pressures fell postnatally, and that this occurred similarly in women with and without fissures. The only significant difference found between the groups was that postnatal constipation was more common in women with fissure (62%) than without (29%), which led the authors to conclude that constipation is the primary cause, and not a secondary effect, of acute postpartum anal fissure.

Management

Acute anal fissures can heal with conservative treatment rather than surgery. In the study by Corby et al (1997), 27 of the 29 cases of postpartum fissure healed without surgery, treatment with stool softeners, laxatives and local anaesthetic cream being given. The other two cases became chronic and were referred for surgical treatment. There are no other studies of postpartum anal fissure but, since chronic anal fissure is relatively common among colorectal outpatient clinic referrals (Banerjee 1997), there are numerous general population based studies on their management.

Surgical treatment, by anal dilation or sphincterectomy, has been found to be successful in healing most chronic anal fissures, but both procedures can result in anal incontinence (Banerjee 1997). These surgical treatments may result in even higher rates of anal incontinence in postpartum women in view of Corby and colleagues' (1997) findings of anal canal pressures being lower anyway after birth. Corby et al (1997) recommended that these surgical procedures should not be used for chronic postpartum anal fissure.

Pharmacological treatments, in particular the use of glyceryl trinitrate (GTN) ointment, have recently been tested in general population studies. When applied to the anus, GTN ointment relaxes the sphincter and leads to a fall in the maximum anal resting pressure, resulting in what is termed a reversible 'chemical sphincterectomy' (Lund et al 1996). Lund & Scholefield (1997) carried out a randomised controlled trial of topical GTN ointment (0.2%) or placebo in 80 general population patients, which showed healing after 8 weeks in 68% of GTN patients compared with 8% of controls. Similar results have been found in other studies, thus the evidence to date suggests that GTN is effective in the treatment of chronic anal fissure. Longer term side effects, however, including headaches and recurrence of symptomatic fissures, have been reported (Carapeti et al 1999, Hyman & Cataldo 1999), and there are no studies of its use in postpartum populations. More recently Brisinda et al (1999) compared topical GTN (0.2%) with botulinum toxin injections in a randomised controlled trial including 50 general population patients, showing healing at 2 months in 60% of the GTN group compared with 96% of the botulinum group. Further research into the efficacy and safety of botulinum injections for the management of anal fissure is necessary, however, before this treatment could be recommended for postnatal women.

FECAL INCONTINENCE

Definition

Fecal incontinence refers to the involuntary passage of bowel contents. The term is usually used to refer to solid or liquid feces, which can be frank incontinence or soiling or staining of underwear, although fecal urgency is often also included. Fecal urgency is where the sensation of needing a bowel movement is felt, but defecation can only be deferred for a short period (a limit of 5 minutes or less is often given). Sometimes flatus incontinence is also included, although anal incontinence would seem a more appropriate term to use to refer to incontinence of both feces and flatus. There is currently no standard definition or classificatory system and no standard forms of questioning, so differences in estimates of incidence and prevalence will occur.

Frequency of occurrence

Childbirth has long been recognised as important in the pathogenesis of fecal incontinence from the histories of old (usually post-menopausal) women presenting in colorectal clinics, but until recent data showed otherwise, it was generally assumed that women rarely (except after a third degree tear) became symptomatic in the postpartum period (Swash 1993). Until recently there had been only a few epidemiological studies specifically investigating the occurrence of postpartum fecal incontinence, but since there has been a rapid increase in studies on this problem, it is described here in some detail. There are also some data on frequency of occurrence from pathophysiological studies of occult anal sphincter injury, and from studies primarily examining other problems (usually urinary incontinence).

Epidemiological studies and trials

Sleep & Grant (1987), in a randomised controlled trial of the effectiveness of pelvic floor exercises on urinary incontinence at 3 months postpartum, reported as an incidental finding that 3% of the women in each of the trial and control groups, experienced 'occasional fecal loss', but this was not mentioned further. Wilson et al (1996), in a study in New Zealand on the prevalence of urinary incontinence at 3 months postpartum, asked about fecal incontinence (new and recurrent symptoms, not including flatus) and found that 73 of the 1505 women (4.9%) experienced this, although no further details were reported.

An observational study in Birmingham, UK of a number of health problems, including fecal incontinence at 10 months postpartum, obtained information on the incidence, duration and nature of this problem in a representative sample of 906 women (MacArthur et al 1997). Research midwives interviewed women in their homes and asked whether they had experienced frank incontinence, soiling or staining of underwear, or urgency (described as 'felt the need to go but couldn't hold on'). There were 36 (4%) women who had experienced one or more of these as a new problem since their delivery, the majority reporting onset as immediate or within the first 2 weeks. A further 2% had recurrent or ongoing symptoms from either a previous birth or because of a pre-existing condition, such as irritable bowel syndrome. Mean symptom duration among the 36 with new symptoms was 23 weeks; only 14 (39%) cases had resolved by the time of interview. Only 5 of the 36 women had consulted their GP about their symptoms.

Zetterström et al (1999), in a prospective study of the incidence of anal incontinence after vaginal delivery among 278 first births in Sweden, found a lower frequency of occurrence than in the previous studies. At 5 months postpartum, 5 women (1.8%) reported incontinence of feces and 70 (25%) of flatus, and at 9 months only 3 (1.1%) reported fecal and 71 (25%) flatus incontinence. A prospective study from Israel also found a lower frequency of fecal incontinence, this time among a general obstetric population (Groutz et al 1999). Among 300 unselected consecutive deliveries inter-viewed at 3 months postpartum, 21 (7%) reported anal incontinence, 2 of whom were incontinent of feces (0.7%), the remainder with incontinence of flatus (6.3%). None had sought medical consultation, despite a quarter regarding the severity of their symptom as moderate or severe. 19 of the 21 symptomatic women were available for a 12 month follow-up, 5 of whom had also had stress urinary incontinence at 3 months. All these 5 remained symptomatic, whilst of the remaining 14, 11 had experienced no further incontinence episodes, the other 3 reporting improvement. Signorello et al (2000), in a retrospective cohort study in the USA designed to examine the effects of midline episiotomy, questioned equal numbers of women who had an episiotomy (n = 205), a tear (n = 204) and an intact perineum (n = 203). At 3 months postpartum the prevalence of fecal incontinence was 2.4% in the intact group, 3.4% after tear and 9.9% after episiotomy. At 6 months the respective proportions were 1.5%, 1.5% and 4.3%, indicating a significant excess in the episiotomy group on both occasions. Flatus incontinence was much more common than fecal incontinence and again there was a significant excess in the episiotomy group (see later). The European longitudinal survey of women's health after childbirth found fecal incontinence rates at 5 months of 1% in Italy and 3% in France, and 3% and 5% respectively at 12 months (Saurel-Cubizolles et al 2000). These health problems were self-reported and no information was given on how fecal incontinence was defined.

Pathophysiological studies

Recently developed investigative techniques, in particular endosono-graphy and manometry, have enabled the imaging of the anal sphincter muscles, and several studies of occult damage to the internal or external anal sphincters have been undertaken, most of which have also obtained data on symptoms. Sultan and colleagues (1993), in a prospective investigation of the antenatal and postnatal occurrence of occult anal sphincter damage, examined 202 women at 34 weeks' gestation, and 150 who returned at 6–8 weeks postpartum. At each assessment the women completed a symptom questionnaire to record anal incontinence, which included fecal and flatus incontinence, and fecal urgency defined as inability to defer defecation for more than 5 minutes. Among the 150 women, 21 (14%) reported postpartum bowel control symptoms: 13 (8.7%) had new symptoms and 8 (5.3%) had recurrent or ongoing ones. These are higher symptom rates than found in the epidemiological studies, probably because agreement to have the anal investigations is more likely in symptomatic women. Greater symptom rates were also found (see below) in similar studies by researchers in Dublin (Donnelly et al 1998, Fynes et al 1999a).

Anal endosonography among the 79 primiparae who delivered vaginally in the study by Sultan et al (1993) showed that none had occult sphincter defects antenatally, but at 6–8 weeks 28 (35%) had defects. Among the multiparae, 19 (40%) had defects antenatally and 22 (44%) at postnatal follow-up. The similar postpartum incidence of defects among the primiparae to the antenatal incidence of defects among multiparae indicates that anal sphincter damage is most likely following the first delivery. All except one of the women with anal incontinence or fecal urgency had a sphincter defect. Sphincter defects, however, were more common than symptoms: only about one third of the women with defects experienced any loss of bowel control. Subsequent studies of anal sphincter damage have had similar findings (Donnelly et al 1998).

Longer term follow-up of women is necessary to determine the extent to which occult sphincter defects have clinical significance. Fynes et al (1999a) prospectively assessed the effects of first and second vaginal deliveries on anal physiology and continence, by following 59 previously nulliparous women through two vaginal deliveries. Ante- and postnatal bowel function questionnaires and assessments of anorectal physiology were completed. Altered fecal continence (including fecal incontinence, urgency and flatus incontinence) was reported by 13 (22%) women after their first delivery, 8 of whom had persistent symptoms during their second pregnancy, 7 of these 8 women having a deterioration of bowel function after the second delivery. 2 of the 13 women had transient symptoms but became incontinent again after the second delivery. In light of these findings, the authors suggested that women with symptomatic large anal sphincter defects should be offered the option of elective caesarean delivery for a subsequent pregnancy.

In total 20 women, one third of the sample, had anal sphincter defects following their first delivery, but only two new defects (both of which were also symptomatic) occurred after the second delivery, confirming the findings of Sultan et al (1993) that the risk of mechanical anal sphincter injury is greatest with the first vaginal delivery. Among the 20 women with primiparous sphincter defects, 7 were asymptomatic, but 3 of these 7 developed symptoms after their second vaginal delivery, whereas only 2 of the 39 women without primiparous sphincter damage went on to develop symptoms (Fynes et al 1999a). It seems therefore that women with symptomless anal sphincter defects after their first delivery are at higher risk of developing fecal incontinence after a second vaginal delivery, although some will still not do so.

Risk factors

Epidemiological and pathophysiological studies are generally in agreement that instrumental delivery is the main factor associated with the occurrence of bowel control symptoms and with occult anal sphincter defects (as well as with third degree tears—see later). In the epidemiological study by MacArthur et al (1997), obstetric data from case notes were obtained, and multivariate analysis showed that forceps and vacuum extraction delivery were the only factors independently associated with new fecal incontinence. In the study of occult sphincter damage by Sultan et al (1993), the only obstetric factor independently associated with this was forceps delivery: 8 of the 10 women delivered by forceps had sphincter defects, although none of 5 delivered by vacuum extraction had defects. There is still a lack of conclusive evidence, however, on the relative effects of instrumental delivery by forceps or vacuum extraction, because the studies that have examined these separately have had only small numbers of either one or both types of instrument.

Donnelly et al (1998), in their Dublin study of sphincter damage, found instrumental vaginal delivery was associated with an 8.1 fold (95% CI 2.7–24.0) risk of anal sphincter injury and a 7.2 fold (95% CI 2.8–18.6) risk of symptoms (urgency, fecal and flatus incontinence). Zetterström et al (1999) in Sweden found a relationship between instrumental delivery and anal incontinence at 5 months postpartum, but not at 9 months. This was an epidemiological study, although a small one, and the authors noted that the instrumental delivery rate among their primiparous sample, at 10%, was very low and may have affected findings on this. Groutz et al (1999) also found a relationship between anal incontinence and instrumental delivery, although again the small sample size makes information on risk factors highly tentative. Almost all of the instrumental deliveries in both these studies were by vacuum extraction. A community based general population study of over 6000 women (median age 58 years) showed that ever having a forceps birth was significantly associated with fecal incontinence (OR 1.5), although how long after the birth this had begun is not known (Assassa et al 2000).

Perineal laceration (except third degree tear) has not been found to be associated with either fecal incontinence symptoms or occult anal sphincter damage. Nor has episiotomy, with two exceptions. One was a type rarely used in the UK for midline episiotomy, and the retrospective cohort design of this study, with a substantial potential for bias, renders findings inconclusive (Signorello et al 2000). The other was in the study by Groutz et al (1999), but this relationship was not independent of instrumental delivery because almost all were accompanied by episiotomy.

Two other independent risk factors of fecal incontinence have been found. Older maternal age was associated with anal incontinence at 5 months and 9 months postpartum in the Swedish study (Zetterström et al 1999). Epidural analgesia was found to be independently associated with bowel control symptoms and with anal sphincter damage by Donnelly et al (1998) in their Dublin study, although Zetterström et al (1999) found no relationship.

The effect of caesarean section delivery in relation to *protecting* against subsequent fecal incontinence is still uncertain. MacArthur et al (1997) found six reports of new fecal incontinence symptoms following 113 emergency sections and none following 61 elective sections, the rate of the former being similar to that following spontaneous vaginal delivery. In the study by Sultan et al (1993) none of the 7 women delivered by elective section, nor the 16 delivered by emergency section, had bowel symptoms or anal sphincter defects, but there was evidence of pudendal nerve neuropathy among the emergency section group. Fynes et al (1998), in a cohort of 34 primiparous women of whom 8 had elective section before labour, 17 had emergency section before 8 cm cervical dilation, and 9 had emergency section after 8 cm dilation, found that none reported alteration in bowel function at 6 weeks, nor was there any evidence of mechanical anal sphincter damage, irrespective of when the section had been performed. Those delivered in late labour, however, even without attempted vaginal delivery, had signs of pudendal nerve damage, which is compatible with the findings of Sultan et al (1993).

There seems to be little evidence of mechanical anal sphincter damage after caesarean section, but damage to the innervation of the anal sphincter can still occur. The main difficulty when attempting to determine the association between caesarean section and fecal incontinence has been that most studies have included relatively few caesarean deliveries, especially when sub-divided according to type. More research on this is required, in particular since it is currently used as evidence by informed women to request elective caesarean section (Al-Mufti et al 1997), about which there has been much ensuing debate (Sultan & Stanton 1996).

Management

Fecal incontinence as an immediate consequence of childbirth, even without tearing of the anal sphincter, is clearly more common than previously suspected, and since few women spontaneously report its occurrence, it is important that midwives specifically ask about bowel control symptoms as part of postnatal care.

Treatment options for non-transient fecal incontinence include conservative therapies as well as surgery. Conservative therapy consists of regulating the stool form using a high fibre diet and antidiarrhoeal agents. Also available are various forms of biofeedback training (Kamm 1998), although evidence on the latter in obstetric cases is mainly available in women with third degree tear (see below). It has been suggested that women with persistent symptoms of loss of bowel control should be reviewed by a colorectal specialist, but this decision will depend on local policy (Cook & Mortensen 1998).

THIRD DEGREE TEAR

Definition

Third degree tear is defined as any tear involving the anal sphincter, although if the anal epithelium is involved some suggest the tear be described as fourth degree (Sultan et al 1995).

Frequency of occurrence and risk factors

Third degree tears have long been known to increase the risk of subsequent fecal incontinence, but this type of trauma as recorded in case notes is uncommon, occurring in 0.5%–1% of vaginal deliveries (Kamm 1998). In a study of a UK hospital population of 8603 vaginal deliveries, 50 (0.6%) were recorded as having third degree tear (Sultan et al 1994). 34 of the 50 women with this trauma agreed to be further investigated and were matched for parity, age and ethnic origin with 88 controls, none of whom had ever had a third degree tear. Anal incontinence (including flatus) or fecal urgency were present in 16 women (42%) with tears and 11 controls (13%). Univariate analysis showed risk factors for third degree tear were forceps delivery, birthweight of over 4 kg, occipitoposterior position at delivery and primiparity (Sultan et al 1994).

A USA study of the incidence and outcome of third degree tear among 16 853 vaginal deliveries found 93 (0.5%) recorded cases; 81 of these were reviewed 3 months after delivery at a colorectal clinic, at which time 16 (20%) suffered from anal incontinence (including flatus) (Walsh et al 1996). Again, univariate analysis showed that third degree tears were significantly more common among primiparae, after forceps delivery, and with heavier infant birthweight. A similar type of study in Adelaide, Australia of 9613 vaginal deliveries over 5 years identified 116 (1.2%) third degree tears (Wood et al 1998). 84 of these were interviewed by telephone, 14 (17%) of whom had fecal or flatus incontinence and 7 had other symptoms of anal dysfunction. Only 3 had consulted any health professional. Primiparity, forceps delivery, episiotomy, birthweight >4000 g and longer second stage labour were all significantly associated, on univariate analysis, with third degree tear.

Management

There is concern about whether third degree tears are correctly identified by doctors and midwives, so that some remain unrecorded; also about the inadequate knowledge of their repair (Sultan et al 1995). Expert opinion suggests that women who have a third degree tear should be prescribed prophylactic laxatives for 2 weeks to prevent constipation and antibiotics to prevent infection. However, prospective studies are required to establish the most appropriate management of these women.

In the case of women who are symptomatic after third degree tear, a recent trial has examined the effects of biofeedback. Biofeedback is a behavioural technique which uses external equipment to demonstrate and alter physiological events using auditory or visual feedback. Standard sensory feedback uses pelvic floor muscle exercises combined with sensory feedback from a perinometer or vaginal cones, and has been used mainly for urinary stress incontinence. This study randomly assigned 36 women symptomatic after recognised anal sphincter tear and 3 after traumatic instrumental delivery, to receive sensory biofeedback (n = 19) or augmented biofeedback (n = 20) (Fynes et al 1999b). The augmented programme included electrical stimulation of the anal sphincter with audiovisual electromyography feedback. After 12 weeks of treatment all women completed a fecal continence questionnaire and had anorectal manometry. Continence scores improved in both groups, but results were better for those who received augmented biofeedback. The study was small with only short term follow-up and more, larger trials are required. In the meantime, however, it does seem that biofeedback can be an effective conservative therapy and the authors suggest it should be commended as first line treatment for symptomatic women.

Secondary anal sphincter repair by colorectal surgery, with varying success rates, can be undertaken for women where conservative treatment has failed (Engel et al 1994).

SUMMARY OF THE EVIDENCE USED IN THIS GUIDELINE

- Several observational studies have shown that all of the postnatal bowel symptoms described in this guideline are relatively common, evidence for fecal incontinence and anal fissure being only recent. Bowel symptoms often occur within the first week or two after delivery and all types have been shown sometimes to persist.

- Conservative treatment of postpartum constipation and haemorrhoids is largely based on current clinical practice.
- One observational study of postpartum acute anal fissure found that almost all cases resolved with conservative treatment of stool softeners, laxatives and local anaesthetic cream.
- Various types of observational studies have shown that fecal incontinence symptoms, occult anal sphincter damage and third degree tears are more common after instrumental deliveries.
- Pathophysiological studies have demonstrated that occult anal sphincter damage occurs after about a third of first vaginal births and rarely after this. Bowel control symptoms are much less common than defects but, if a defect occurs, symptoms after subsequent vaginal deliveries are more likely.
- Various small studies suggest that caesarean section delivery reduces the risk of fecal incontinence since mechanical anal sphincter damage does not seem to occur; but it does not prevent incontinence because neurological damage can still occur. Larger studies and further research on this, especially of elective sections, is required.
- There is consensus that third degree tears confer an increased risk of fecal incontinence, but since these tears are rare, many women with fecal incontinence will not have had this type of trauma.
- There is consensus that women do not spontaneously report bowel control symptoms, but if asked (as shown in studies) will disclose the information.

WHAT TO DO

INITIAL ASSESSMENT

- Ask if bowels opened since delivery.
- Ask about specific difficulties to enable identification of the following: constipation, haemorrhoids, anal fissure, loss of bowel control, including soiling, faecal urgency and flatus incontinence.
- Check from delivery records if the woman sustained a third degree tear.
- Ascertain history of bowel problems
  - pre-existing bowel condition, e.g. irritable bowel syndrome, ulcerative colitis
  - bowel problems associated with pregnancy or previous delivery.

CONDITIONS WHICH REQUIRE IMMEDIATE REFERRAL TO GP

- Severe, swollen haemorrhoids which cannot be replaced in anal canal.
- Frank incontinence of faeces.

CONSTIPATION

- Establish duration of constipation, whether this occurred in pregnancy, and if it was a common problem prior to pregnancy.
- Check any medication the woman is taking for side effects of constipation. If iron supplementation is being taken, check the most recent Hb result to see if it can be discontinued.
- Give advice on adequate dietary fibre and fluid intake.
- If these measures do not resolve the constipation and the woman is uncomfortable, a prescription for a laxative (expert opinion suggests lactulose), should be obtained from the GP. Expert opinion suggests glycerine suppositories should be used as the next line of management if the woman still has not had her bowels opened within 4–5 days of taking lactulose. This should be discussed with the woman and, if she agrees with this treatment, administer the suppositories in accordance with prescription regulations. Review the following day. If the woman feels that the constipation has still not resolved, discuss this and refer to the GP.
- Constipation is associated with anal fissure (see later) so be alert for this, particularly if the woman reports severe pain or blood loss on defecation.

HAEMORRHOIDS

- It is appropriate to assess the perianal area to confirm a diagnosis and degree of haemorrhoids since other symptoms, in particular anal fissure or blood loss following the passing of a hard stool, could be misdiagnosed as 'haemorrhoids'.
- Ask about onset (ante- or postnatal) and severity. Explain that haemorrhoids are common, and that conservative treatment is usually appropriate. Women should be advised that haemorrhoids may bleed following a bowel movement, but a woman who experiences *painful* bleeding may have an anal fissure, and this should be checked (see below).

- All women should be advised to avoid/treat constipation with dietary fibre and by obtaining a prescription for a laxative (lactulose) if dietary measures do not resolve constipation.

- If on examination the haemorrhoid is purple, severe, swollen and can not be manually returned to the anal canal, *urgent GP referral should be made.* A woman may have a less acute, thrombosed haemorrhoid which may not require immediate GP referral, but expert opinion suggests if advice has been taken and it does not resolve within 2 weeks GP referral should be made.

- If less severe haemorrhoids, and conservative measures have been followed but it remains uncomfortable, refer to the GP.

- If painful, topical applications of haemorrhoid creams (i.e. Anusol) may provide some pain relief. This can be bought from the pharmasist.

- If the woman reports persistent bleeding after initial treatment for haemorrhoids, she should be referred to her GP for clinical assessment.

ANAL FISSURE

- The woman will report severe pain on defecation, blood loss and constipation and may have had a sudden onset.

- Conservative treatment should be pursued initially; advise about dietary and fluid intake to prevent and/or treat constipation with stool softeners or laxatives. The woman may obtain temporary relief from topical application of Anusol, which can be bought from the pharmacist.

- If unresolved refer to the GP for prescription of glyceryl trinitrate (GTN) ointment, but inform the woman of possible side effects.

- If after 2 weeks from commencing GTN treatment symptoms remain severe, expert opinion suggests referral back to the GP for possible clinical referral.

FECAL INCONTINENCE/URGENCY/SOILING/FLATUS

- If the woman has loss of bowel control, determine if this is flatus, urgency (not being able to defer a bowel movement), soiling or staining of underwear or frank incontinence. If frank incontinence of liquid or solid stool, refer to GP immediately.

- Ask about symptoms of constipation (if constipation is severe, incontinence may be due to overflow). If overflow is suspected, referral should be made to the GP for advice about treatment owing to the potential severity of constipation.

- If the woman reports soiling, check if this is associated with other bowel problem. If not, advise re constipation and refer to the GP if unresolved after 2 weeks.

- If the woman reports urgency or flatus incontinence that bothers her, expert opinion suggests referral to the GP after 2 weeks.

- Review regularly. GP referral should be made after discussion with the woman. Women with severe incontinence may require referral to a colorectal surgeon for possible secondary repair.

THIRD DEGREE TEAR

- Women who have a third degree tear should have their perineum examined at regular intervals to ensure that the wound is healing. If no healing progress within 2 weeks, expert opinion suggests referral to the GP.

• Check that the woman is taking adequate pain relief, which should be paracetamol. If this is not easing pain, refer to the GP for stronger analgesia.

• Ask if laxative (lactulose) was prescribed for the woman when she was discharged home. If it was, advise on the importance of adhering to the prescription to avoid constipation. If not, refer to the GP for a prescription. Ideally the woman should take this for 2 weeks.

• Advice on dietary intake of fibre and fluids should also be stressed especially if stronger analgesia has been prescribed. If constipation is severe and/or the woman is uncomfortable, referral to the GP should be made.

• Stress the importance of perianal hygiene and if there are concerns about infection of the tear, referral should be made to the GP.

GENERAL ADVICE

• Advise that it is common not to have a bowel motion for 24–48 h after delivery.

• It is important to stress an adequate intake of fluid and dietary fibre, so that the need for laxatives will be less likely. Laxatives may produce mild abdominal cramps.

• If discomfort from perineal trauma is experienced, adequate analgesia should be taken prior to opening bowels. Paracetamol is the drug of choice: analgesia containing codeine may exacerbate constipation.

• If anxious about passing a bowel motion for the first time after delivery, reassure that this is highly unlikely to result in further perineal damage. It may feel more comfortable if a clean sanitary towel is held against the perineum when passing a motion.

SUMMARY GUIDELINE

BOWEL PROBLEMS

INITIAL ASSESSMENT

- Ask if/when bowels opened since delivery
- Identify specific difficulties (constipation, haemorrhoids, anal fissure, fecal incontinence)
- Check if there is third degree tear
- Ascertain relevant history, e.g. pre-existing bowel conditions

IMMEDIATE REFERRAL TO THE GP IS REQUIRED IF:

- Severe, swollen haemorrhoid which cannot be replaced in anal canal
- Frank fecal incontinence

WHAT TO DO

CONSTIPATION

- Check history and current medication
- Advise dietary intake of fibre and fluids
- If not resolved get prescription for lactulose
- If still not resolved after 4–5 days get prescription for glycerine suppositories
- If still not resolved and if uncomfortable, refer to GP

HAEMORRHOIDS

- Assess degree of haemorrhoid
  - severe prolapsed haemorrhoid immediate GP referral
  - third degree (prolapsed but can be replaced manually) —if advice taken and not resolved in 2 weeks refer to GP
  - first/second degree (less severe)—if advice taken but remains uncomfortable refer to GP
- Recommend Anusol to all
- Dietary and other advice to avoid/treat constipation
- If woman reports persistent bleeding after initial treatment refer to GP

ANAL FISSURE

- Dietary and other advice to avoid/treat constipation
- Anusol cream
- If not resolved refer to GP for GTN ointment
- If not resolved within further 2 weeks refer back to GP

FECAL INCONTINENCE

- Frank incontinence—refer to GP immediately
- Urgency/flatus—if not resolved within 2 weeks refer to GP
- If soiling ascertain presence of other bowel problems and treat as appropriate
- If not advise re constipation and if not resolved within 2 weeks refer to GP

THIRD DEGREE TEAR

- Examine perineum regularly to check healing and ensure adequate pain relief
- Check lactulose and antibiotics have been prescribed
- Stress importance of perianal hygiene
- Assess perianal healing and severity of pain
- If no healing progress within 2 weeks or pain persistent refer to GP

GENERAL ADVICE

- It is common not to have a bowel motion for a few days after delivery
- Advise on high fibre diet and adequate fluid intake
- If there is perineal pain, recommend analgesia (paracetemol) before attempting to pass a motion
- It may feel more comfortable if a clean maternity pad is held against the perineum when passing a motion

REFERENCES

Al-Mufti R, McCarthy A, Fisk N M 1997 Survey of obstetricians' personal preference and discretionary practice. Eur J Obstet Gynecol Reprod Biol 73: 1–4

Assassa L P, Dallosso S, Perry C et al and the Leicestershire MRC Incontinence Study Team 2000 The association between obstetric factors and incontinence: a community survey. Br J Obstet Gynaecol 107: 822

Banerjee A K 1997 Treating anal fissure (editorial). BMJ 314: 1638–1639

Brisinda G, Maria G, Bentivoglio A R et al 1999 A comparison of injections of botulinum toxin and topical nitroglycerin ointment for the treatment of chronic anal fissure. N Engl J Med 341(2): 65–69

Brown S, Lumley J 1998 Maternal health after childbirth: results of an Australian population based survey. Br J Obstet Gynaecol 105: 156–161

Carapeti E A, Kamm M A, McDonald P J et al 1999 Randomised controlled trial shows that glyceryl trinitrate heals anal fissures, higher doses are not more effective, and there is a high recurrence rate. Gut 44(5): 727–730

Cook T A, Mortensen N J M 1998 Management of faecal incontinence following obstetric injury. Br J Surg 85: 293–299

Corby H, Donnelly V S, O'Herlihy C et al 1997 Anal canal pressures are low in women with postpartum anal fissure. Br J Surg 84(1): 86–88

Donnelly V S, Fynes M, Campbell D et al 1998 Obstetric events leading to anal sphincter damage. Obstet Gynecol 92(6): 955–961

Engel A F, Kamm M, Sultan A H et al 1994 Anterior anal sphincter repair in patients with obstetric trauma. Br J Surg 81: 1231–1234

Fynes M, Donnelley V S, O'Connell P R et al 1998 Cesarean delivery and anal sphincter injury. Obstet Gynecol 92(4): 496–500

Fynes M, Donnelly V S, Behan M et al 1999a Effect of second vaginal delivery on anorectal physiology and faecal continence: a prospective study. Lancet 354: 983–986

Fynes M M, Marshall K, Cassidy M et al 1999b A prospective, randomized study comparing the effect of augmented biofeedback with sensory biofeedback alone on fecal incontinence after obstetric trauma. Dis Colon Rectum 42(6): 753–761

Garcia J, Marchant S 1993 Back to normal? Postpartum health and illness. In: Robinson S, Tickner V (eds) Research and the midwife. Conference proceedings 1992. University of Manchester

Glazener C M A, Abdalla M I, Stroud P et al 1995 Postnatal maternal morbidity: extent, causes, prevention and treatment. Br J Obstet Gynaecol 102: 282–287

Groutz A, Fait J B, Lessing M P et al 1999 Incidence and obstetric risk factors of postpartum anal incontinence. Scand J Gastroenterol 34: 315–318

Hardwick R H, Durdey P 1994 Should rubber band ligation of haemorrhoids be performed at the initial outpatient visit? Ann R Coll Surg Engl 76(3): 185–187

Hibbard B M 1988 Principles of obstetrics. Butterworths, London

Hooker G D, Plewes E A, Rajgopal C et al 1999 Local injection of bupivacaine after rubber band ligation of hemorrhoids: prospective, randomized study. Dis Colon Rectum 42(2): 174–179

Hyman N H, Cataldo P A 1999 Nitroglycerin ointment for anal fissures: effective treatment or just a headache? Dis Colon Rectum 42(3): 383–385

Jewell D J, Young G 2000 Interventions for treatment of constipation in pregnancy. Cochrane Review 3. The Cochrane Library, Oxford

Johanson J F, Rimm A 1992 Optimal nonsurgical treatment of haemorrhoids: a comparative analysis of infrared coagulation, rubber band ligation, and injection sclerotherapy. Am J Gastroenterol 87(11): 1600–1606

Kamm M A 1998 Faecal incontinence. BMJ 316: 528–532

Lund J N, Scholefield J H 1997 Glyceryl trinitrate is an effective treatment for anal fissure. Dis Colon Rectum 40(4): 468–470

Lund J N, Armitage N C, Scholefield J H 1996 Use of glyceryl trinitrate ointment in the treatment of anal fissure. Br J Surg 83: 776–777

MacArthur C, Lewis M, Knox E G 1991 Health after childbirth. HMSO, London

MacArthur C, Bick D E, Keighley M R B 1997 Faecal incontinence after childbirth. Br J Obstet Gynaecol 104: 46–50

MacRae H M, McLeod R S 1995 Comparison of haemorrhoidal treatment modalities: a meta-analysis. Dis Colon Rectum 38(7): 687–694

Pfenninger J L 1997 Modern treatments for internal haemorrhoids. BMJ 314: 1211–1212

Saurel-Cubizolles M-J, Romito P, Lelong N et al 2000 Women's health after childbirth: a longitudinal study in France and Italy. Br J Obstet Gynaecol 107: 1202–1209

Shelton M G 1980 Standardised senna in the management of constipation in the puerperium—a clinical trial. South African Med J 57: 78–80

Shepherd J 1997 Helping women to cope with pregnancy changes. In: Sweet B (ed) Mayes' midwifery. Baillière Tindall, London, ch 20

Signorello L B, Harlow B L, Chekos A K et al 2000 Midline episiotomy and anal incontinence: retrospective cohort study. BMJ 320: 86–90

Sleep J, Grant A 1987 Pelvic floor exercises in postnatal care—the report of a randomised controlled trial to compare an intensive exercise regimen with the programme in current use. Midwifery 3: 158–164

Sultan A H, Stanton S L 1996 Preserving the pelvic floor and perineum during childbirth—elective caesarean section? Br J Obstet Gynaecol 103: 731–734

Sultan A H, Kamm M A, Hudson C N et al 1993 Anal-sphincter disruption during vaginal delivery. N Engl J Med 329(26): 1905–1911

Sultan A H, Kamm M A, Hudson C N et al 1994 Third degree obstetric anal sphincter tears: risk factors and outcome of primary repair. BMJ 308: 887–891

Sultan A H, Kamm M A, Hudson C N 1995 Obstetric perineal trauma: an audit of training. J Obstet Gynaecol 15: 19–23

Swash M 1993 Faecal incontinence—childbirth is responsible for most cases. BMJ 307: 636

Tramonte S M, Brand M B, Mulrow C D et al 1997 The treatment of chronic constipation in adults: a systematic review. J Gen Intern Med 12(1): 15–24

Walsh C J, Mooney E F, Upton G J et al 1996 Incidence of third-degree perineal tears in labour and outcome after primary repair. Br J Surg 83(2): 218–221

Wilson P D, Herbison R M, Herbison G P 1996 Obstetric practice and the prevalence of urinary incontinence three months after delivery. Br J Obstet Gynaecol 103: 154–161

Wood J, Amos L, Rieger N 1998 Third degree anal sphincter tears: risk factors and outcome. Aust N Z J Obstet Gynaecol 38(3): 414–417

Zetterström J P, López A, Anzén B et al 1999 Anal incontinence after vaginal delivery: a prospective study in primiparous women. Br J Obstet Gynaecol 106: 324–330

7

Depression and other psychological morbidity

INTRODUCTION

Psychological disturbances following childbirth vary in timing of onset, duration and severity. Three main conditions are generally described: the 'blues', depression and puerperal psychosis (Kendall-Tackett & Kantor 1993), although the extent to which they are interrelated is not clear (Hannah et al 1992). This guideline deals mainly with depression as the most common manifestation of significant postpartum psychological morbidity. Although postnatal blues are more widely experienced, this is a transient condition and generally of minor importance. Puerperal psychosis is rare, but is serious and requires urgent referral for treatment, so must be recognised by the midwife. Other less common psychological conditions which may be experienced by postpartum women, in particular stress reactions, anxiety disorders and disorders of the mother–infant relationship, will not be referred to in this guideline.

There is increased concern that much psychiatric morbidity around the time of childbirth remains unidentified. The recent *Report on confidential enquiries into maternal deaths in the United Kingdom 1994–1996* (Department of Health 1998) included, for the first time, a chapter on maternal deaths associated with psychiatric illness; 18 deaths were attributed to psychiatric illness within the first year of delivery.

POSTNATAL DEPRESSION

Definition

Postnatal depression, although sometimes difficult to define and recognise, was described in a classic study by Pitt in 1968 as: 'what lies between the extreme of severe puerperal depression, with the risk of suicide and infanticide, and the trivial weepiness of "the blues"; something occurring frequently, much less dramatic than the former, yet decidedly more disabling than the latter' (Pitt 1968, p. 1325). There is no precise definition of postnatal depression, but its clinical features are similar to depression occurring at any time within the general population and include lethargy, tearfulness, oversensitivity, hopelessness, anxiety, guilt, irrational fears and disturbed sleep patterns. The typical gradual onset means that it may not be easily distinguishable from the fatigue and emotional lability experienced by most mothers as they recover from childbirth and adjust to the demands of the baby (Holden 1991).

Frequency of occurrence

The frequency of depression after childbirth has been well documented in observational studies which have found a prevalence range of 10–15%, the variation due to different assessment times and diagnostic criteria (Cooper et al 1988, Cox et al 1982, Kumar & Robson 1984). Case register studies show that the number admitted to hospital with postnatal depression is low, much less than 1% of all women delivered (Kendall et al 1987). Not all postnatal depression is identified by, or reported to, health professionals, so that the proportion who receive treatment from the primary health care team is probably somewhere between these two figures.

The onset and duration of postnatal depression are not clearly defined since most studies have been cross-sectional, assessing prevalence at various points in time. Cooper et al (1988) carried out a prospective investigation of postpartum psychiatric disorder in a group of 483 women who booked into an Oxford maternity unit, with comprehensive assessments undertaken antenatally and at 3, 6 and 12 months postpartum. The proportions of new onset cases at each postpartum assessment were 7.7%, 5.2% and 2.2%, making an incidence over the whole 12 months of about 15%. A quarter of cases had started within the first postpartum month. Duration was often quite short, two thirds of cases lasting for 3 months or less. This study, as well as others, however, has shown that some women can experience depression after childbirth which persists for longer than this (Romito 1990).

Although the term postnatal depression is commonly used by professionals and by mothers, some researchers have questioned the extent to which it comprises a specific entity (Green 1998). In the study by Cooper et al (1988) described above, similar psychiatric data were also obtained from a group of 313 non-puerperal women available from a general population sample in Edinburgh. Data from all women aged 16–40 who had had no pregnancy or delivery in the previous 12 months were compared with the postpartum sample. This comparison led the authors to conclude that there were no differences in the prevalence or nature of non-psychotic psychiatric disorder among postpartum and non-puerperal groups of women. Cox et al (1993) also compared a group of postnatal women with controls who were neither pregnant nor had had a baby in the previous 12 months. In this study the controls were from the same community and were individually matched for age, marital status and number of children. A threefold higher rate of depression within 5 weeks of childbirth was found amongst the postnatal women, compared with the equivalent time period for control women. At 6 months postpartum, however, the prevalence of depression was similar in both groups (9.1% in the postnatal group; 8.2% in the control group). Cox et al (1993) concluded that the threefold excess within the first month is most likely as a result of the 'life event' of giving birth and the immediate impact of a new family member; and that the category of postnatal depression remains a useful diagnostic term. Whether or not the prevalence, duration and nature of depression after childbirth is similar to that occurring among women generally, its appearance after birth remains relevant to those involved in providing maternity services.

Risk factors

In the search for possible risk factors for postnatal depression, studies have examined a large number of maternal, obstetric and socio-demographic characteristics, in particular obstetric interventions, age, parity, marital status, psychiatric history, interpersonal relationships and hormone disorders. Given the range of samples, timings and instruments of assessment used in studies it is not surprising that conclusions have been contradictory. However, one undisputed risk factor, found by all those studies in which it has been examined, is the reporting of a poor (or absent) relationship with the partner (Romito 1990). A personal or family history of psychiatric disorder has also been identified as a strong risk factor for postpartum depression in numerous studies (Watson et al 1984), although not all have found this association (Kumar & Robson 1984, Murray et al 1995). Hormonal links with postnatal depression have generally not been found (Romito 1990).

Additional effects

A positive association between maternal physical health and postpartum recovery and maternal emotional wellbeing in an Australian study of 1336 women, followed up at 6–7 months postpartum, has recently been documented (Brown & Lumley 2000). The Edinburgh Postnatal Depression Scale (EPDS) was used to assess emotional wellbeing with a score of ≥ 13. Similar associations were shown in a more in-depth telephone interview of a sub-sample of women at 7–9 months.

Postnatal depression may have longer term consequences for the development of the child. Prospective studies have found an association between maternal mood disorder and cognitive development at age 4–5, especially among children of socio-economically disadvantaged mothers (Coghill et al

1986, Sharp et al 1995), and insecure infant attachment at age 18 months (Murray 1992). Cooper & Murray (1998), in a clinical review of postnatal depression, proposed that the association between postnatal depression and adverse child development was as a consequence of an impaired pattern of communication between the woman and her infant. That postnatal depression might have a lasting impact on a woman and her infant highlights the importance of the early detection and management of this problem.

Management

The management of postnatal depression will depend on its severity, but can consist of pharmacological treatments, directive and non-directive counselling and support visits from relevant health professionals, including community psychiatric nurses and health visitors. Treatment may comprise a 'package' of these. For a small proportion of women, admission to a specialised unit will be necessary. The effects of treatment of postnatal depression, however, have only been assessed in a few small randomised controlled trials. There are two Cochrane systematic reviews of treatment for postnatal depression (Lawrie et al 2000, Ray & Hodnett 2000).

Ray & Hodnett (2000) reviewed the effects of professional and/or social support interventions for women with postnatal depression. They identified only two trials which involved 137 women. In one of the trials (Holden et al 1989), the intervention was provided by health visitors who had received training in non-directive counselling and made weekly half-hour visits to the women in the treatment group for 8 weeks. The women in this study had been identified as depressed by screening with the Edinburgh Postnatal Depression Scale (EPDS) at 6 weeks, and by psychiatric interview at 12 weeks postpartum. 55 of the 60 women identified agreed to participate, and at 25 weeks postpartum 31% of those in the treatment group compared with 62% in the control group had still not fully recovered (OR 0.29, 95% CI 0.10–0.86). In the other trial (Appleby et al 1997), the effectiveness of cognitive–behavioural counselling and fluoxetine (for effects of fluoxetine see below) was examined in a factorial design randomised controlled trial which Ray & Hodnett (2000), in their Cochrane review, recategorised in order to assess the effects of the counselling. The counselling intervention comprised six sessions with a psychologist who had received brief training in cognitive–behavioural therapy. At 15 weeks postpartum there was a significantly reduced incidence of depression in the counselled, compared with the non-counselled group (OR 0.37, 95% CI 0.13–0.99). In view of the small numbers, however, the reviewers consider the conclusions to be tentative, with larger trials being required, not only to obtain more evidence on the effects of support in treating depression, but also to consider it as a preventive strategy and to determine which form of support is most effective.

The other Cochrane review (Lawrie et al 2000) assessed the benefits of oestrogens and progestogens for the prevention and treatment of postnatal depression. This review was based on two trials, both concerning treatment (not prevention) which included a total of 241 women. One trial (Lawrie et al 1998) randomised 180 South African women to receive a single dose of norethisterone enantate (synthetic progestogen) or placebo given within 48 hours of delivery and lasting 8–12 weeks. Progestogen was associated with significantly *more* depression at 3 months postpartum than placebo, leading the reviewers to conclude that there is no place for synthetic progestogens in the treatment of postnatal depression. The reviewers also note that in view of this increased depression rate, any long-acting progestogen contraceptives should be used with caution in the postnatal period. The other trial of hormonal treatment carried out in London (Gregoire et al 1996) randomised 61 women with major depression that had begun within 3 months of birth to receive transdermal beta-estradiol or placebo. Mean depression scores using the EPDS were found to be lower in the treatment group (13.3) than the control group (16.5). The reviewers concluded that high dose oestrogen therapy may be of modest benefit in severe postnatal depression but were concerned that the trial groups may not have been sufficiently comparable. The reviewers found no trials of hormonal treatment to *prevent* postnatal depression, nor any trials of progesterone therapy in treating postnatal depression.

One of the trials of the effects of cognitive–behavioural therapy, as noted above, also examined the effects of fluoxetine, an antidepressant (Appleby et al 1997). It found that the effects of the antidepressant and the cognitive–behavioural counselling were equivalent, and that there was little additional benefit from receiving both treatments.

SCREENING FOR POSTNATAL DEPRESSION USING THE EDINBURGH POSTNATAL DEPRESSION SCALE

The Edinburgh Postnatal Depression Scale (EPDS) (Cox et al 1987, see p. 141) was developed as a screening instrument acceptable to women who may not have considered themselves to be depressed. The scale originally included 13 items, although following a validation study (Cox 1986), it became apparent that it could be reduced to 10 items without impairing its effectiveness as a screening tool. The items were validated in a counselling intervention study on a sample of 84 women (Cox et al 1987). The authors originally intended that the EPDS should be administered at the 6–8 week postnatal check, but in practice it was apparent that this would fail to identify some depressed women, as the onset of depression can occur after this (Cox et al 1993). Cox (1996), in a description of the development of the EPDS, recommended three screening times within the first 6 months to maximise the detection of postnatal depression: at 5–6 weeks, 10–14 weeks and 20–26 weeks. There is little evidence, however, of whether this guidance for screening is adhered to in practice.

The EPDS has been administered at various different times in both observational studies and randomised controlled trials; the variation in the timing of administration has not affected the scale's validity (Brown & Lumley 1998, Gerrard et al 1993, Holden et al 1989). Currently the EPDS is used in routine practice mainly by health visitors, although it was designed for use by other members of the primary health care team, including midwives and GPs.

Scoring the EPDS is straightforward. Each of the 10 items has four possible responses and the woman is asked to choose the response that comes closest to how she has felt during the previous 7 days. The responses are then scored. A score of 12 or more is considered to identify those women more likely to have depression (Cox et al 1987). The questionnaire has been found to be acceptable to both women and health professionals and is quick to complete (Holden 1991).

The EPDS was not designed as a diagnostic instrument, but to be used as a first line screening tool, followed by a standardised psychiatric interview by a psychiatrist or GP to make the decision to diagnose and/or treat. The scale has been found to have high sensitivity and specificity (Cox et al 1987, Harris et al 1989). A large community study found a sensitivity of 88% and a specificity of 92.5% (Murray & Carothers 1990) (sensitivity is the proportion of women with depression correctly identified by the scale and specificity is the proportion of women who *do not* have depression correctly identified by the scale).

It is important to emphasise in using the EPDS that clinical judgement and common sense on the part of the health professionals should always override an EPDS score.

POSTPARTUM BLUES

The transient and frequent experience of weepiness and mood instability is known as the postpartum blues (Romito 1990). It is a syndrome experienced a few days after the delivery, typically between about the third and tenth days. The exact definition of the blues varies to some extent (Kennerley & Gath 1989, O'Hara et al 1991), but the most commonly reported symptoms include tearfulness, lability of mood, irritability, and sometimes headache (Hannah et al 1992, O'Hara et al 1991, Piper 1992, Snaith 1983). Observational studies have found the prevalence of the blues to range from 50 to 80% (George & Sandler 1988, Kendall et al 1981, Stein et al 1981). They are considered to be self limiting and no specific treatment is required, although reassurance is sometimes needed. Studies have found evidence of a higher incidence of the blues among women who suffer from postnatal depression (Beck et al 1992, O'Hara et al 1991), although a plausible hormonal basis to account for this link has not been identified (Murray 1992, O'Hara et al 1991).

PUERPERAL PSYCHOSIS

The most severe form of postnatal psychiatric morbidity is puerperal psychosis; it is also the most uncommon. It is characterised by thought disorders and/or severe depression and may even result in suicide or infanticide. Although very rare, as noted earlier, deaths from suicide were included in the most recent *Report on confidential enquiries into maternal deaths* (Department of Health 1998). Four of these deaths occurred within 42 days of delivery, the other 14 deaths after this, but within the first postnatal year. Some of the women had a previous history of psychiatric problems or substance abuse. The midwife's role is particularly important in the early recognition of severe psychiatric disturbance, as these symptoms must be managed quickly and appropriately.

The prevalence of psychotic illness in the puerperium is about 1 in 500 births (Godfroid & Charlot 1996). Protheroe (1969) found that 94% of puerperal psychosis had an onset within 4 weeks of childbirth, 65% within 2 weeks. A sudden onset, after an interval of wellbeing since the birth, is characteristic (Riley 1995, Snaith 1983, Thurtle 1995). It is an atypical illness which may be characterised by schizophrenic and affective symptoms (Riley 1995). Clinically the woman may complain of a confusing mixture of symptoms and may have no insight into the fact that she is mentally ill. A range of presenting symptoms are described by Riley (1995) and include restlessness, distractibility, being over-active and over-talkative, with racing thoughts and 'flight of ideas'. The mother may express grandiose ideas and become irritable or even violent if these are thwarted, and may believe that her baby is dead or deformed. The woman may be disorientated in time, place and person and could later complain of partial or complete amnesia for the period of the illness (Piper 1992, Riley 1995).

Hospitalisation is usually necessary and it is preferable to admit the woman and her infant together to a specialist unit. Tranquillisers are often indicated as a matter of urgency, to control disturbed and restless behaviour and ensure sleep. Where drugs are ineffective in acceptable dosages, electro-convulsive therapy (ECT) may occasionally be used to control symptoms (Riley 1995). ECT was developed initially as a treatment for schizophrenia and a Cochrane systematic review which included 12 trials of this in general (not postpartum) populations found that when added to treatment with antipsychotic medication, there was a significant increase in symptom resolution, although the effect did not persist (Tharyan 2000). Side effects of ECT such as amnesia, however, have been reported

(Robinson 1998). Further research is required of the most appropriate management of childbirth related psychosis.

POSTNATAL DEBRIEFING

There has been much recent discussion in midwifery journals and textbooks about whether there is a need to 'debrief' women of their labour and delivery experiences in order to prevent psychological morbidity (Abbott et al 1997, Ralph & Alexander 1994), although there is limited evidence of the appropriateness of this (Alexander 1998, 1999). Debriefing generally involves the promotion of a form of emotional 'catharsis' by encouraging recollection of the traumatic event. It is often offered as an intervention following serious incidents to prevent post-traumatic stress disorder (PTSD), although a recent Cochrane systematic review has shown no evidence from non-postpartum populations that psychological debriefing is useful for the prevention of PTSD after traumatic incidents (Wessely et al 2000). Two randomised controlled trials have investigated debriefing in a postnatal population (Lavender & Walkinshaw 1998, Small et al 2000). In the first, 120 postnatal primigravidae in a UK maternity unit were allocated to receive a 'debriefing session' with the research midwife (n = 56) or not (n = 58). The intervention provided by the midwife, who was not a trained counsellor, whilst still on the postnatal ward, consisted of an interview during which women could spend as much time as they needed (range 30–120 minutes) talking about their labour, asking questions and discussing their feelings. The Hospital Anxiety Scale (HAD) was the main outcome measure, administered by postal questionnaire 3 weeks after delivery. Controls compared with women who received the intervention were more likely to have a high HAD anxiety score (OR 13.5, 95% CI 4.1–56.9) or HAD depression score (OR 8.5, 95% CI 2.8–30.9). Since the HAD scale has not been validated for use in the postnatal period however, and the definition of a high score in the analysis was different from that used to calculate sample size, results should be interpreted with caution. Wessely (1998), in a commentary which appeared in the same journal issue as the paper, considered that given the timing of debriefing and follow-up at 3 weeks postpartum, it was more likely to have been the transient state of postpartum dysphoria (blues) that was affected by the intervention rather than postnatal depression. Small et al (2000) in a large well-designed Australian trial among 1041 women who had operative delivery found no significant differences in depression and overall health status at 6 months postpartum of the group allocated to midwife de-briefing. Proportionate differences in scores however, which were worse for the intervention group, led the authors to conclude that the possibility that debriefing contributed to emotional health problems for some women could not be excluded.

SUMMARY OF THE EVIDENCE USED IN THIS GUIDELINE

- Numerous observational studies have shown depression to occur in the postpartum period in about 10–15% of women.
- There is an increased risk of postnatal depression where there is a poor relationship with the partner or the mother is unsupported and in women with a previous psychiatric history, but there is a lack of consensus on other risk factors.
- Use of screening instruments, in particular the EPDS, will enable the early detection of women who may be experiencing postnatal depression.
- Evidence from two small randomised controlled trials suggests that simple forms of psychological intervention—non-directive counselling and cognitive–behavioural counselling—may reduce the incidence and duration of postnatal depression, but larger trials are required.
- There is probably a modest benefit of oestrogen in the management of severe postnatal depression. Progestogen is associated with increased rates of depression. Long-acting progesterone based contraceptives, therefore, should not be prescribed for women during the immediate postnatal period.
- Evidence of the effects of 'supportive' listening as debriefing in preventing postnatal depression indicates that it is likely to be of no benefit.

WHAT TO DO

INITIAL ASSESSMENT IF WOMAN HAS DEPRESSION

The main role of the midwife in relation to postpartum psychiatric morbidity is to be alert to its detection.

- Ask how the woman is feeling; is she anxious about anything; how does she feel about the baby and being a mother; is she able to sleep?
- Ask her about support from her partner, relatives or friends.
- *Be especially alert if:*
  - there is a history of psychiatric illness
  - her relationship with the partner is difficult or she is unsupported
  - what appeared to be the blues does not resolve.

In addition to being alert to the detection of psychological conditions, it is necessary to be able to distinguish the various manifestations. The table below sets out the main features of the blues, depression and psychosis.

Main features of postpartum blues, postnatal depression and puerperal psychosis, with action for midwife

	Postpartum blues	Postnatal depression	Puerperal psychosis
Frequency	50–80%	10–15%	1 in 500
Symptoms	Tearfulness; irritability; lability of mood; sometimes headache	Lethargy; tearfulness; over-sensitivity; hopelessness; anxiety; guilt; irrational fears; disturbed sleep patterns	Thought disorders; delusion; confusion; agitation; fear; insomnia; severe depression. Rarely suicide/infanticide
Onset	Few days after delivery. Typically between 3 and 10 days	Mainly within first month or two of delivery	Most commonly in first 4 weeks after delivery
Duration	A few days or less	Most resolve within about 3 months or less, especially with treatment, but can persist	Variable
Action	Transient condition. No action except reassurance needed unless does not resolve	If suspected (either from consultation or EPDS screening) refer to GP and liaise with health visitor	**Contact GP for immediate home visit. Do not leave woman alone. Explain to family**

If at any time the midwife suspects the existence of any other psychological morbidity, such as severe anxiety disorders or stress reactions, the woman should be referred to the GP.

WOMAN SHOWING SYMPTOMS OF DEPRESSION

- Where there is concern that a woman may be suffering from postnatal depression, following discussion with the woman, GP referral should be made, and the health visitor informed. The midwife should liaise closely with the GP and health visitor to plan care.

- Immediate referral should be made if the midwife is concerned there is a risk of suicide or child abuse.

- Encourage her to utilise support of partner (and/or close relative or friend) in helping care for the baby and in talking about her feelings.

- Ensure that the woman knows how to contact the midwife and/or health visitor whenever she needs to.

- Offer literature on self-help and details of local and/or national support groups.

- If at any time the midwife suspects that the woman may be suffering from other psychiatric morbidity such as severe anxiety disorder or stress reactions, she should be referred to the GP, with degree of urgency dependent on severity.

WOMAN SHOWING SYMPTOMS OF PUERPERAL PSYCHOSIS

- Contact GP immediately for home visit.
- Do not leave the woman alone.
- Explain the situation to the woman and partner.

INTRODUCTION OF THE EPDS INTO PRACTICE

Before considering the introduction of EPDS screening, it is important that consultation with all of the relevant members of the primary health care team takes place to establish current practice, timing of administration of the scale and availability and access to mental health services, should a woman require this. A policy for the use of the EPDS should be agreed by all relevant health professionals. Efforts should be made to ensure training needs of those health professionals who will administer the scale are identified.

HOW TO ADMINISTER THE EPDS

The EPDS (below) should be completed by all women to screen for depression, using locally agreed protocols. Copies of the EPDS and instructions in its use are given. The scale should be administered by the midwife and/or the health visitor and management of women with high scores should be agreed, including follow-up. The following strategy is consistent with the recommendations of Cox et al (1987), Holden (1994).

- With a score of 8 or less, reassure the woman that no potential depression problem has been identified. *No further action is needed unless the midwife notes that the mother has any evidence at all of mental disorder.*

- With a score of 9–11, discuss this with the woman and offer to contact the health visitor for her. Explain that the health visitor may be able to offer her extra support in the form of 'listening visits'. If there is any doubt about or concern that the woman is depressed, GP referral is necessary.

- With a score of 12 or more refer to the GP for further assessment and offer to contact the health visitor.

- *It is important to emphasise that clinical judgement and common sense should always override an EPDS score.*

THE EDINBURGH POSTNATAL DEPRESSION SCALE (EPDS)

The EPDS consists of 10 statements which relate to symptoms of postnatal depression but is not a complete checklist of depressive symptoms. The woman is asked to underline the reply which comes closest to how she has been feeling over the past week. All information is confidential.

Instructions

- All ten items must be completed by the woman

- The EPDS is a *self report* scale, so only in exceptional circumstances should the professional need to help the woman in its completion

- The woman should be encouraged to complete the scale without discussing her answers with others, as this may influence her response

- Scores for individual items range from 0–3 according to severity. For most questions a positive answer for the first option scores 3. For items marked* the first option scores 0 and the fourth option 3. The total score is calculated by adding the scores for each of the 10 items. Please refer to the guideline for appropriate action to take after the scores have been added up.

Please complete:

Woman's name: . . . .

Address: . . . .

. . . .

Baby's age (in weeks): . . . .

Today's date: . . . .

Health visitor: . . . .

General practitioner: . . . .

As you have recently had a baby, we would like to know how you are feeling now. Please UNDERLINE the answer which comes closest to how you have felt **IN THE PAST WEEK**, not just today.

1. I have been able to laugh and see the funny side of things:
   * As much as I always could
   Not quite so much now
   Definitely not so much now
   Not at all

2. I have looked forward with enjoyment to things:
   * As much as I ever did
   Rather less than I used to
   Definitely less than I used to
   Hardly at all

3. I have blamed myself unnecessarily when things went wrong:
   Yes, most of the time
   Yes, some of the time
   Not very often
   No, never

4. I have been worried or anxious for no very good reason:
   * No, not at all
   Hardly ever
   Yes, sometimes
   Yes, very often

5. I have felt scared or panicky for no very good reason:
   Yes, quite a lot
   Yes, sometimes
   No, not much
   No, not at all

6. Things have been getting on top of me:
   Yes, most of the time I haven't been able to cope at all
   Yes, sometimes I haven't been coping as well as usual
   No, most of the time I have coped quite well
   No, I have been coping as well as ever

7. I have been so unhappy that I have had difficulty sleeping:

    Yes, most of the time

    Yes, sometimes

    Not very often

    No, not at all

8. I have felt sad or miserable:

    Yes, most of the time

    Yes, quite often

    Not very often

    No, not at all

9. I have been so unhappy that I have been crying:

    Yes, most of the time

    Yes, quite often

    Only occasionally

    No, never

10. The thought of harming myself has occurred to me:

    Yes, quite often

    Sometimes

    Hardly ever

    Never

(From Cox et al 1987 and Holden 1994)

SUMMARY GUIDELINE

DEPRESSION AND OTHER PSYCHOLOGICAL MORBIDITY

INITIAL ASSESSMENT

- Ask how the woman is feeling; is she anxious; disappointed with the baby/maternal experience; unable to sleep
- Ask her about support from partner, relatives, friends
- Be especially aware if
  - there is a history of psychiatric illness
  - her relationship with her partner is difficult or she is unsupported
  - what appeared to be the blues does not resolve

IMMEDIATE REFERRAL TO GP IS REQUIRED IF:

- Woman showing symptoms of puerperal psychosis
- Woman who midwife considers to be at risk of suicide or child abuse

WHAT TO DO

WOMAN SHOWING SYMPTOMS OF DEPRESSION

- If concerned that a woman may be depressed, discuss this and refer to GP and inform health visitor
- Encourage support of partner (and/or close relative or friend) in caring for baby
- Ensure that she knows how to contact the midwife and/or health visitor at any time
- Offer self-help and support group literature
- If at any time the midwife suspects the existence of any other psychological morbidity, such as severe anxiety disorders or stress reactions, the woman should be referred to the GP

The summary below sets out the main features of the blues, depression and psychosis, and action to be taken by midwife.

	Postpartum blues	Postnatal depression	Puerperal psychosis
Frequency	50–80%	10–15%	1 in 500
Symptoms	Tearfulness; irritability; lability of mood; sometimes headache	Lethargy; tearfulness; over-sensitivity; hopelessness; anxiety; guilt; irrational fears; disturbed sleep patterns	Thought disorders; delusion; confusion; agitation; fear; insomnia; severe depression. Rarely suicide/infanticide
Onset	Few days after delivery. Typically between 3 and 10 days	Mainly within first month or two of delivery	Most commonly in first 4 weeks after delivery
Duration	A few days or less	Most resolve within about 3 months or less, especially with treatment, but can persist	Variable
Action	Transient condition. No action except reassurance needed unless does not resolve	If suspected (either from consultation or EPDS screening) refer to GP and liaise with health visitor	**Contact GP for immediate home visit. Do not leave woman alone. Explain to family**

EPDS – flow chart summary

Use to screen all women for PND
(check local protocols)

**If concerned about the woman's psychological
wellbeing regardless of EPDS score, refer to GP**

Score 8 or less
Reassure woman
No action needed if showing no evidence of
mental disorder

Score 9–11
Ask about concerns
Offer to contact health visitor
Refer to GP if there are any concerns

Score 12 or more
Ask about concerns
Dispel negative feelings
Advise re support groups
Give literature
Offer to contact health visitor
Refer to GP

REFERENCES

Abbott H, Bick D E, MacArthur C 1997 Health after birth. In: Henderson C, Jones K (eds) Essential midwifery. Mosby, London, ch 14

Alexander J 1998 Confusing debriefing and defusing postnatally: the need for clarity of terms, purpose and value. Midwifery 14(2): 122–124

Alexander J 1999 Can midwives reduce postpartum psychological morbidity? A randomised controlled trial. MIDIRS comments. MIDIRS Midwifery Digest 9(3): 370–371

Appleby L, Warner R, Whitton A et al 1997 A controlled study of fluoxetine and cognitive–behavioural counselling in the treatment of postnatal depression. BMJ 314: 932

Beck C T, Reynolds M A, Rutowski P 1992 Maternity blues and postpartum depression. JOGGN 21(4): 287–293

Brown S, Lumley J 1998 Maternal health after childbirth: results of an Australian population based survey. Br J Obstet Gynaecol 105: 156–161

Brown S, Lumley J 2000 Physical health problems after childbirth and maternal depression at six to seven months postpartum. Br J Obstet Gynaecol 107: 1194–1201

Coghill S, Caplan H, Alexandra H et al 1986 Impact of maternal postnatal depression on cognitive development of young children. BMJ 292: 1165–1167

Cooper P J, Murrary L 1998 Postnatal depression. Clinical review. BMJ 316: 1884–1886

Cooper P J, Campbell E A, Day A et al 1988 Non psychotic psychiatric disorder after childbirth. A prospective study of prevalence, incidence, course and nature. Br J Psychiatry 152: 799–806

Cox J L 1986 Postnatal depression: a guide for health professionals. Churchill Livingstone, Edinburgh

Cox J 1996 Origins and development of the 10-item Edinburgh Postnatal Depression Scale. In: Cox J, Holden J (eds) Perinatal psychiatry. Gaskell, Glasgow, pp 115–124

Cox J L, Connor Y, Kendell R E 1982 Prospective study of the psychiatric disorders of childbirth. Br J Psychiatry 140: 111–117

Cox J L, Holden J M, Sagovsky R 1987 Detection of postnatal depression. Development of the 10-item Edinburgh Postnatal Depression Scale. Br J Psychiatry 150: 782–786

Cox J L, Murray D, Chapman G 1993 A controlled study of the onset, duration and prevalence of postnatal depression. Br J Psychiatry 163: 27–31

Department of Health 1998 Why mothers die. Report on confidential enquiries into maternal deaths in the United Kingdom 1994–1996. The Stationery Office, London

George A, Sandler M 1988 Endocrine and biochemical studies in puerperal mental disorders. In: Kumar R, Brockington I F (eds) Motherhood and mental illness. Wright (Butterworths), Cambridge, vol 2, pp 78–81

Gerrard J, Holden J M, Elliot S A et al 1993 A trainer's perspective of an innovative training programme to teach health visitors about the detection, treatment and prevention of postnatal depression. J Adv Nurs 18: 1825–1832

Godfroid I O, Charlot A 1996 Postpartum psychiatry. Rev Med Brux 17(1): 22–23

Green J M 1998 Postnatal depression or perinatal dysphoria? Findings from a longitudinal community-based study using the Edinburgh Postnatal Depression Scale. J Reprod Infant Psychol 16(2/3): 143–155

Gregoire A J P, Kumar R, Everitt B et al 1996 Transdermal oestrogen for the treatment of severe postnatal depression. Lancet 347: 930–933

Hannah P, Adams D, Lee A et al 1992 Links between early post-partum mood and post-natal depression. Br J Psychiatry 160: 777–780

Harris B, Huckle P, Thomas R et al 1989 The use of rating scales to identify post-natal depression. Br J Psychiatry 154: 813–817

Holden J M 1991 Postnatal depression: its nature, effects and identification using the Edinburgh Postnatal Depression Scale. Birth 18(4): 211–221

Holden J 1994 Using the Edinburgh Postnatal Depression Scale in clinical practice. In: Cox J, Holden J (eds) Use and misuse of the Edinburgh Postnatal Depression Scale. Royal College of Psychiatrists, London, ch 9

Holden J M, Sagovsky R, Cox J L 1989 Counselling in general practice setting: controlled study of health visitor intervention in treatment of postnatal depression. BMJ 298: 223–226

Kendall R E, McGuire R J, Connor Y et al 1981 Mood changes in the first three weeks after childbirth. J Affect Disord 3: 317–326

Kendall R E, Chalmers J C, Platz C 1987 Epidemiology of puerperal psychosis. Br J Psychiatry 150: 662–673

Kendall-Tackett K, Kantor G K 1993 Postpartum depression. A comprehensive approach for nurses. Sage, London

Kennerley H, Gath D 1989 Maternity blues: 1. Detection and measurement by questionnaire. Br J Psychiatry 155: 356–362

Kumar R, Robson K M 1984 A prospective study of emotional disorders in childbearing women. Br J Psychiatry 144: 35–47

Lavender T, Walkinshaw S A 1998 Can midwives reduce postpartum psychological morbidity? A randomised trial. Birth 25(4): 215–219

Lawrie T A, Hofmeyr G J, de Jager M et al 1998 A double-blind randomised controlled trial of postnatal norethisterone enanthate: the effect on postnatal depression and serum hormones. Br J Obstet Gynaecol 105: 1082–1090

Lawrie T A, Herxheimer A, Dalton K 2000 Oestrogens and progestogens for preventing and treating postnatal depression. Cochrane Review 3. The Cochrane Library, Oxford

Murray L 1992 The impact of postnatal depression on child development. J Child Psychol Psychiatry 33: 543–561

Murray L, Carothers A D 1990 The validation of the Edinburgh Postnatal Depression Scale on a community sample. Br J Psychiatry 157: 288–290

Murray D, Cox J L, Chapman G et al 1995 Childbirth: life event or start of a long term difficulty? Br J Psychiatry 166: 595–600

O'Hara M W, Schlechte J A, Lewis D A et al 1991 Prospective study of postpartum blues. Arch Gen Psychiatry 48: 801–806

Piper M 1992 Emotional and mental disturbances of the puerperium. Midwives Chronicle & Nursing Notes (August): 228–235

Pitt B 1968 "Atypical" depression following childbirth. Br J Psychiatry 114: 1325–1335

Protheroe C 1969 Puerperal psychoses: a long term study. Br J Psychiatry 115(518): 9–30

Ralph K, Alexander J 1994 Borne under stress. MIDIRS Midwifery Digest 4(3): 330–332

Ray K L, Hodnett E D 2000 Caregiver support for postnatal depression. Cochrane Review 3. The Cochrane Library, Oxford

Riley D 1995 Perinatal mental health: a source book for health professionals. Radcliffe Medical Press, Oxford

Robinson J 1998 Sinister stories. Br J Midwifery 6(5): 334

Romito P 1990 Postpartum depression and the experience of motherhood. Acta Obstet Gynecol Scand 69: suppl 154

Sharp D, Hay D, Pawlby S et al 1995 The impact of postnatal depression on boys' intellectual development. J Child Psychol Psychiatry 36: 1315–1337

Snaith R P 1983 Pregnancy related psychiatric disorder. Br J Hosp Med 29: 450–456

Stein G, Marsh A, Morton J 1981 Mental symptoms, weight change and electrolyte excretion during the first postpartum week. J Psychosom Res 25: 395–408

Tharyan P 2000 Electroconvulsive therapy for schizophrenia. Cochrane Review 3. The Cochrane Library, Oxford

Thurtle V 1995 Post-natal depression: the relevance of sociological approaches. J Adv Nurs 22: 416–424

Watson J P, Elliott S A, Rugg J et al 1984 Psychiatric disorder in pregnancy and the first postnatal year. Br J Psychiatry 144: 453–462

Wessely S 1998 Commentary: reducing distress after normal childbirth. Birth 24(4): 220–221

Wessely S, Rose S, Bisson J 2000 Brief psychological interventions ("debriefing") for immediate trauma related symptoms and the prevention of post-traumatic stress disorder. Cochrane Review 3. The Cochrane Library, Oxford

8

Fatigue

INTRODUCTION

Fatigue is a non-specific symptom shown in general population studies to be experienced at some time by many people. Women in these studies commonly report higher rates of fatigue than men (Chen 1986, Cox et al 1987, David et al 1990). It is a well recognised problem anecdotally after childbirth, and although few studies have specifically investigated this, it has been reported as widespread and persistent (Bick & MacArthur 1995, Brown & Lumley 1998, Glazener et al 1995, MacArthur et al 1991). These studies found that fatigue was underreported to health professionals, as women expect to experience it when caring for a new baby and consider it to be a normal reaction to the physiological changes of childbirth. However, it is likely that the duration and severity of postnatal fatigue will determine whether for some women it has a significant effect on their health (Rubin 1975).

Definition

The simplest definition of fatigue is probably that of the physiologist—a decrease in response after prolonged activity (Welford 1953). Fatigue is a protective mechanism whereby the body slows down or stops so that overuse is prevented and regeneration can take place. No direct correlation has been described between the level of fatigue experienced and energy expenditure or stress. Individual coping style, physical fitness, psychological make-up and motivation may mean that one person will feel fatigued when others do not (Hart et al 1990). Fatigue is primarily a subjective experience, incorporates psychological and environmental factors and is to be expected in certain situations: after excessive physical exertion, or following prolonged wakefulness without adequate sleep. The difficulty in classification of fatigue as abnormal or excessive is compounded following childbirth, when care of an infant inevitably results in increased activity and disturbed sleep patterns. One definition of fatigue used widely in nursing research is that of the North American Nursing Diagnosis Association (NANDA): 'An overwhelming sustained sense of exhaustion and decreased capacity for physical and mental work' (Lee et al 1994, Milligan & Pugh 1994, NANDA 1990, Piper 1994).

Frequency of occurrence

Various instruments to measure subjective fatigue have been developed, for example, Symptom Distress Scale, Yoshitake's Fatigue Scale, Rhoten Fatigue Scale, Pearson Byars Fatigue Feeling Tone Scale, but none has gained widespread acceptance as a standard objective measure of fatigue (Hart et al 1990). The most common method of documenting prevalence of fatigue in studies of postpartum women is a tick box response to a question asking whether the women have experienced fatigue or extreme tiredness, usually within a list of symptoms.

The wording of this question will influence the morbidity identified. The question may be worded to establish whether the symptom is new, with scope to record previous experience of the symptom, onset in relation to the birth, duration, and whether medical help had been sought and received (MacArthur et al 1991). Asking women about health symptoms which have been a problem will elicit positive responses only from those who do not assume some degree of the problem to be normal after childbirth (Brown & Lumley 1998). Questions worded to establish point prevalence without attempting to determine if this is a new symptom will include those whose symptoms predate childbirth and exclude those whose symptoms have resolved (Saurel-Cubizolles et al 2000). Importance is sometimes assessed in postpartum studies by relating rates of fatigue to those for other health symptoms after childbirth, but attribution of cause and effect in cross-sectional data is impossible (Gardner & Campbell 1991).

High rates of fatigue are to be expected, and have been reported in the early postpartum period. Early studies, of small numbers of women, described high rates of concern about fatigue among women at 4 and 6 weeks postpartum (Fawcett & York 1986, Gruis 1977). Tulman & Fawcett (1988) found that, of 70 women who had delivered a full term infant within the previous 5 years only 51% of women reported that they had regained their usual level of energy by 6 weeks postpartum. The authors suggested that the traditional view of recovery from childbirth being complete at 6 weeks postpartum needed to be reconsidered. This was a small study where the sampling method limits generalisability: the majority of women were recruited at a conference for members of a caesarean section prevention movement. In another small qualitative study, Ruchala & Halstead (1994) also found that at 2 weeks after discharge from hospital, 76% of 50 postpartum women interviewed cited fatigue as a major physical concern. Fatigue was an underlying theme for the women, and being tired was a major descriptor of their postpartum experiences for 44% of the women.

The first broad-based sample to describe persistence of fatigue and other health problems well beyond 6 weeks was by MacArthur et al (1991). In a West Midlands study of over 11 000 women, questioned 1–9 years after they had given birth, 17.1% of women reported extreme tiredness, as they perceived it, occurring within 3 months of delivery and lasting for more than 6 weeks: 12.2% of the women had not experienced tiredness this extreme before. For 6.1% of the sample, the fatigue had persisted for more than a year. The association between childbirth and persistent fatigue was confirmed in a further, more detailed study, which necessitated shorter recall (Bick & MacArthur 1995). Of 1278 women surveyed at 6–7 months after delivery, 41% reported extreme tiredness occurring *for the first time* within 3 months of the delivery and lasting for over 6 weeks. The majority of these women reported the symptoms of fatigue as persistent.

Similar findings were described by Glazener et al (1995), in a prospective observational study of a 20% sample (n = 1249) of women who delivered in one year in the Grampian region of Scotland. Women were surveyed about health problems at discharge from hospital, at 8 weeks and, for half of the sample, again at 12–18 months postpartum. Tiredness was reported by 42% of women at discharge, 59% up to 8 weeks and 54% between 2 and 18 months postpartum. In an Australian study of health among 1336 women delivered in 1993 and surveyed at 6–7 months postpartum, 69.4% reported tiredness/exhaustion occurring as a problem some time since the birth (Brown & Lumley 1998). A postal questionnaire survey for the Audit Commission (Garcia et al 1998), of a sample of 2406 women throughout England and Wales at 4 months postpartum, asked about health problems as part of a wider study of maternity care. The women were asked to think back to 10 days, 1 month and 3 months and say which of a number of health problems they had at those times: 43% reported having had fatigue at 10 days, 31% at 1 month and 21% at 3 months. None of these studies attempted to establish whether the symptoms reported were new in the postpartum period.

Recall of between 6 weeks and 9 years was required in these studies but the findings are consistent with those from a recent prospective study estimating point prevalence of various health problems at 5 months and 12 months postpartum (Saurel-Cubizolles et al 2000). In a recent longitudinal survey of the health of 697 Italian and 589 French women delivered in 1993/94, tiredness was reported by 46.1% Italian and 48.4% French women at 5 months postpartum. By 12 months these figures had increased to 60.7% and 67.5% respectively.

These assessments have been able to determine only the presence or absence of fatigue, with some attempt to delineate its duration. In a Canadian study Smith-Hanrahan & Deblois (1995) used the Rhoten Fatigue Scale (a visual analogue scale ranging from not tired to totally exhausted) to measure present fatigue intensity in subjects reporting fatigue at 2–3 days, 1 week and 6 weeks postpartum. The aim of the study was to examine the effect of early discharge on maternal fatigue and ability to perform activities of daily living, but difficulties experienced in enacting the randomisation mean that comparisons between arms in this study are unlikely to be valid. For the study population as a whole, however, some level of fatigue was recorded on the Rhoten scale in 95% of the 81 mothers at the time of discharge from hospital. At 6 weeks postpartum, this figure was 86%. Sufficient detail is not given in the paper to determine the overall proportion with severe tiredness at each assessment point, but it appears to be around 20% of all women.

Self-reported fatigue is entirely subjective but objective measures are not available. In a study designed to examine the extent, severity and effect of postnatal symptoms, fatigue was commonly reported (Bick & MacArthur 1995). Of 1278 women who completed a postal questionnaire, 523 (40%) reported fatigue, and of these 77% (n = 405) reported that it impacted on their lives in some way. Women reported that fatigue affected their ability to concentrate, they felt bad-tempered or did not want to socialise. Interestingly, it did not appear to affect their ability to care for their infant. Postnatal fatigue was associated with problems related to resuming sexual intercourse in the 8 weeks and 12–18 months follow-up of women who participated in the study of postnatal health in the Grampian region (Glazener 1997). All of these surveys will be subject to some degree of response bias. In addition, such studies have limited ability to place the person's reported level of fatigue within their physical, psychological, work and social context. In studies where more detailed evidence of fatigue was sought, or where a more multidimensional view of fatigue was explored, the small size and non-random sampling methods used limit their generalisability (Gardner 1991).

Finding an appropriate comparison group to determine if fatigue prevalence is higher in postpartum women than in other groups is complex. Gjerdingen & Froberg (1991) compared adoptive mothers (6 weeks after adoption) and biological mothers (7 weeks after delivery) with a nonpregnant control group who had attended for pelvic examination. Both adoptive and biological mothers reported more fatigue than controls but the generalisability and validity of the comparison is very limited. Of 444 women with a mean age of 38 attending a general practice in London, 12% were suffering from 'chronic fatigue' (David et al 1990). Of the 167 men in the study (mean age 41), the figure was 9%. Sampling methods and the predominantly middle class composition of the sample limit generalisability of these findings. In a Norwegian population-based random sample of 3500 people, 11.4% of all women (aged 19–80 years) reported substantial fatigue lasting 6 months or longer (Loge et al 1998). In a US survey of a national probability-based sample of adults aged 25–74 years (the size of the sample and response rates are not quoted) 20.4% of women reported suffering from fatigue, compared to 14.3% of men.

Risk factors

Pugh & Milligan (1993) categorised potential factors in predisposing a woman to childbearing fatigue as physical, psychological and situational. Physical factors may be normal physiological changes or pathological ones, which in the postpartum period can include effects of mode of delivery, anaemia, infection and haemorrhage (Chen 1986, Paterson et al 1994). Psychological factors might include the mother's reaction to childbearing, and mental states such as anxiety and depression. Situational factors may be personal, such as parity, age, method of feeding and sleep patterns, or environmental, including socio-economic status, social support and lifestyle.

Physical risk factors

Delivery factors identified in the study by MacArthur et al (1991) as independent risk factors for long term fatigue included multiple pregnancy, longer first stage of labour, inhalation anaesthesia and postpartum haemorrhage, but not operative delivery. Milligan et al (1990) did show a significant association between caesarean section and fatigue in a group of 259 women surveyed before discharge from hospital, but when the same women were surveyed at 6 weeks and 3 months no significant effect was seen. Findings from the other two large studies previously quoted are consistent with an early excess for caesarean section which diminishes over time. At 12–18 months fatigue was not associated with caesarean section in Glazener's study, but there was an association in the reports of fatigue at 0–13 days and at up to 8 weeks (Glazener et al 1995). Tiredness was more common in women delivered by caesarean section and surveyed at 6–7 months in Brown & Lumley's (1998) study but the effect was not statistically significant (Brown & Lumley 1998). The other studies have not reported on the other delivery factors.

Few studies have examined the physiological determinants of postnatal fatigue, but Paterson et al (1994) investigated the impact of a low (<10.5 g/dl) haemoglobin (Hb) on the postnatal mental and physical health of 1010 women. Hb results were obtained at 'booking', 34 weeks, third day post delivery and at 6 weeks postpartum. Women were asked to complete questionnaires about their health at 10 days, 4 weeks and 6 weeks after delivery. Full data including Hb were obtained from only 52% of the original sample. A low Hb on day 3 was more likely to be diagnosed in younger women (aged under 25); among primiparae; women who had had operative or instrumental delivery; women who had a low Hb at 34 weeks' gestation; and those with a blood loss of over 250 ml recorded at delivery. Some of these variables are interrelated (for example parity and mode of delivery), but statistical analysis to determine independence of effect was not undertaken. Women with a low Hb at day 3 were significantly more likely to report feeling low in energy in the questionnaire at day 10. They were also more likely to report being breathless, faint and dizzy, and to have painful sutures and tingling of the fingers or toes. By 6 weeks no difference was apparent between groups with and without low Hb, but it is not clear from the paper what action was taken on the basis of the Hb result, though it is apparent that some of the women in the study were taking iron supplements.

Other physical problems worth considering if a woman reports extreme tiredness are infections and, though much less common, thyroid disorders and cardiomyopathy (Atkinson & Baxley 1994). Chronic fatigue syndrome (CFS), a condition where persistent fatigue is felt and significant disability experienced without apparent cause, may affect women after childbirth, but no studies have reported rates of occurrence in this group. In a general population study of fatigue, Chen (1986) found heavier women more likely to be fatigued than lighter ones (based on Body Mass Index).

Psychological risk factors

Fatigue is a well recognised symptom of depression though it may be difficult to clarify whether anxiety and depression are the cause or result of fatigue (Unterman et al 1990). Of 1065 postpartum women who reported depression in MacArthur et al's (1991) study, 47% (496) also reported extreme tiredness. These 496 women constituted 35% of all women (1427) who reported extreme tiredness. In Brown & Lumley's (1998) survey of 1336 Australian women at 6–7 months postpartum, tiredness was 3.4 times more likely to be reported by women with scores on the Edinburgh Postnatal Depression Scale indicating probable depression.

Gardner (1991) collected data by questionnaire at 2 days, 2 weeks and 6 weeks postpartum from 68 non randomly selected American women. The sample were only mildly fatigued, as scored on the Rhoten Fatigue Scale, and fatigue and depression scores were significantly, but not strongly, correlated at 2 days and 2 weeks, but not at 6 weeks postpartum. Milligan et al (1990) found that comparatively little of the variation in fatigue at 6 weeks and 3 months postpartum was explained by other factors in models which controlled for depression.

The correlation between fatigue symptoms and psychiatric disorder has also been demonstrated in studies of patients with chronic fatigue syndrome. In a nested case control study, 60% of 214 chronic fatigue patients were found to have a current psychiatric disorder compared to 19% of 214 matched controls (Wessely et al 1996).

It is not possible to determine cause and effect in cross-sectional studies and no cohort studies were found. One prospective study of 63 women was designed to investigate the relationship between sleep disruption prior to birth, during labour and in the early postpartum period, and the subsequent development of the postnatal blues (Wilkie & Shapiro 1992). The findings suggested that a night time labour and a history of sleep disturbance in late pregnancy may influence development of postnatal blues.

Situational risk factors

There have been contrasting findings with regard to a possible association between fatigue and parity. MacArthur et al (1991) found fatigue more common in older primiparae. Glazener et al (1995) and Brown & Lumley (1998) found no association with parity and did not report on an effect of age. In Gardner's small study (n = 35), older women reported less fatigue but the sample selection, response rate and overall low levels of fatigue in this study diminish its generalisability and power (Gardner 1991).

The method of infant feeding may have an impact on postnatal fatigue. Two studies found breastfeeding more likely to be associated with fatigue than bottle feeding (MacArthur et al 1991, Milligan & Pugh 1994). In a small non-random convenience sample, breastfeeding problem severity was associated with fatigue in each assessment at 3 days and 3, 6 and 9 weeks postpartum (Wambach 1998).

With the trend in earlier discharge from hospital a few small studies have attempted to explore the effect of earlier postpartum discharge on women's health. In their qualitative study, Ruchala & Halstead (1994) link comments that several women made about hospital stay being too short with the importance of fatigue underlying many issues. Smith-Hanrahan & Deblois (1995) attempted to randomise 125 women into early and 'traditional' discharge groups and to compare fatigue levels at three intervals in the first 6 weeks postpartum. Implementation was found to be impractical as 29 of 67 women randomised to receive traditional care were discharged early due to bed shortages. The study, subject to other methodological weaknesses, was analysed in three groups, but no differences in fatigue levels were demonstrated. Using a rest and activity questionnaire, Carty et al (1996) failed to show a difference in fatigue at 1 and 4 weeks postpartum between women discharged in 3 days or sooner and those who stayed in hospital longer.

Oakley (1992) proposed that changes in the social circumstances of women during the last decade, such as increasing number of lone parent families, lack of support, and the need to continue in paid employment, were likely to lead to fatigue in the new mother. MacArthur et al (1991) showed higher reports of extreme tiredness in unmarried women. In the European survey women were asked to describe their relationship with their partner. At 12 months postpartum, rates of extreme tiredness in lone mothers in both countries were lower than in all cohabiting groups except those who described their relationship as very good

(Saurel-Cubizolles et al 2000). It has been suggested that diversity of social support can act as a buffer to the stress of maternal fatigue on parenting (Parks et al 1992).

Classification of socio-economic status in postpartum women is difficult and little evidence of an effect on postpartum fatigue has been shown. Among the 35 women in Gardner's (1991) study, fatigue at 6 weeks postpartum was negatively correlated with the mother's education level but, as mentioned earlier, the generalisability of these results is limited for reasons discussed above. In Saurel-Cubizolle et al's (2000) study tiredness at 12 months postpartum was reported more frequently by women with a severe financial problem though only for French women was the difference statistically significant (70.5 vs 60.9 p <0.02). Tiredness was reported more often for women employed at 12 months postpartum in this study, though again the effect was statistically significant only for French women (70.5% vs 60.9%).

Management

Fatigue is common postpartum, but it is also a major feature of many illnesses. It is important that any medical conditions associated with fatigue should be identified and treated. In Paterson et al's (1994) study of postpartum anaemia, as well as symptoms of fatigue at 10 days, women with a low Hb at day 3 were more likely to report being breathless, faint and dizzy, and to have painful sutures and tingling of the fingers or toes. Slightly more women with a low Hb at day 3 scored 14 or more on the EPDS at day 10 (10% vs 7%), but this excess was not statistically significant. It does suggest that symptom assessment and EPDS results may be of use in discriminating physiological causes of fatigue. Anaemia in postpartum women may remain undetected, as many obstetric units do not perform routine postnatal Hb. Predictors of low postpartum Hb in Paterson et al's study have already been quoted and could help in diagnosing anaemia as a cause of postpartum fatigue.

Given the strong association between fatigue and anxiety and depression, it is important to exclude psychological illness in fatigued patients.

In the absence of a physical or psychological cause for postpartum fatigue, it is widely assumed that nothing can be done. No studies of effectiveness of management strategies for postpartum fatigue were found. Some literature exists in relation to the management of chronic fatigue syndrome (CFS), but since a major component of this disorder is significant disability without apparent cause, applicability to postpartum women is limited (Fulcher & White 1997, Price & Couper 2000). The appropriateness of applying this to postpartum women is questionable when disability is not a feature and an evident cause for the fatigue experienced can be seen in the requirements of caring for one or more babies.

Management strategies for fatigue can be broadly divided into those where sufferers are advised to limit the demands placed on their bodies and those geared around a graded increase in activity. The strategy of limiting demand amounts to treating fatigue as a protective symptom against overstressing the body. In trying to increase activity, the association between inactivity and increased levels of fatigue is assumed to be causal (Chen 1986).

Strategies suggested for the management of fatigue are not specific to postpartum women and draw on data, often qualitative, from studies of fatigued patients with serious medical illnesses such as cancer or on no data at all (Hart et al 1990, Piper 1994). Nonetheless, in the absence of good evidence of effective management, some of the recommendations from these papers are included.

Given the strong association between fatigue and psychological factors, therapeutic listening, counselling and patient education to reduce anxiety and increase sense of control are proposed (Piper 1994).

Hart et al (1990) suggest management should be based on the individual being able to influence her own health, and that she should have an active role in decisions about treatment. By increasing the mother's awareness of the possible problems of the puerperium, she can be advised on changing behaviour to overcome or minimise the effects of fatigue, for example by taking a rest after feeding the infant. A small study of 14 women suggests that breastfeeding in the side-lying position resulted in lower fatigue as measured on a modified fatigue symptoms checklist (Milligan et al 1996).

To help people recognise sources of excessive energy consumption, it is suggested that they maintain a fatigue diary for one week (Hart et al 1990). Recording a detailed diary may not be feasible for postpartum women but it might well help for them to review their activities with a view to conserving energy.

The importance of sleep seems superfluous to state but Hart et al (1990) point out the body's requirement for sleep in maintaining function. Rest is suggested as a means of conserving or restoring energy. Several short periods of rest are postulated to be more beneficial than one long period. This latter method of intervention is more realistic for the postpartum mother, who is likely to be able to find short periods to rest rather than a long period. Symptoms of fatigue may reflect underlying marginal nutritional deficiency (Hart et al 1990), and the importance of a well balanced diet should be discussed, particularly with lactating mothers. Calorific intake is also important.

Exercise has been associated with improvement in mood, level of tension, anxiety, psychological functioning and depression whilst physical deconditioning may be caused by reduced physical activity, which may accentuate physical and psychological effects (Fulcher & White 1997). Achieving an appropriate pattern of activity and rest is problematic in the postpartum woman and energy needs to be conserved. It may be that in the immediate postnatal period exercise should be limited to maintenance of function and support of daily activities.

Natural techniques for relieving fatigue are also discussed by Hart et al (1990). These include progressive muscle relaxation, acupressure, reflexology, massage, relaxation imagery and visualisation, but further evidence is required of their benefit for postnatal women.

SUMMARY OF THE EVIDENCE USED IN THIS GUIDELINE

- Fatigue is a non-specific symptom assessed subjectively. General population studies show that it is common but prevalence rates are high among postpartum women.
- In the absence of a standard objective measure of fatigue, prevalence among postpartum women has usually been ascertained by asking women about this as one of many postnatal health problems.
- Observational studies of self-reported postnatal health problems show that for many women fatigue can become a chronic symptom, and for some it will affect other aspects of their lives.
- It is important to identify and manage any underlying psychological or physical illness that may present with fatigue.
- Advice on how to incorporate adequate rest periods into their daily routine and how to ensure they maintain adequate nutritional intake may help women to reduce their fatigue levels.

WHAT TO DO

INITIAL ASSESSMENT

• Exclude depression. Symptoms to be aware of are: lethargy; tearfulness; anxiety; guilt; irritability; disturbed sleep patterns; lack of energy; poor appetite; poor concentration. If depression is suspected refer to guideline 7 on Depression and Other Psychological Morbidity.

• Exclude anaemia. Ask about breathlessness, dizziness, tingling in fingers and toes. Check haemoglobin level. If low treat as local policy.

• Consider and exclude possibility of infection, thyroid disorder or other physical or medical problems. If any are identified use appropriate guideline if available or refer to GP.

• If there are no underlying conditions give general advice as below.

'SIMPLE' FATIGUE

• Help the woman plan her time each day to include short periods of rest. It may be appropriate to suggest that she asks a relative or friend to help with household tasks so that she has more time to spend caring for her baby.

• Explain the importance of exercise. Advise a short walk each day at a time when the mother feels she has most energy, which should then be followed by a short period of rest.

• Check that dietary intake is adequate and stress the need to eat at regular intervals.

• Where appropriate discuss social circumstances and lifestyle (e.g. young single mother). If the woman feels it necessary, referral to a health visitor may be arranged, if additional social support would be beneficial.

• Encourage the woman to discuss any problems or worries she may have with the midwife and/or a close friend or family member.

• If the woman is breastfeeding suggest that she use the side-lying position for at least some of the feeds.

• It may be helpful if the woman keeps a 'diary' of daily tasks for 1 week to assess if fatigue is related to any particular activity or time of day. Her activities can then be reviewed in relation to this.

• Review symptoms at subsequent visits.

• *Refer to GP if concerned about wellbeing at any time.*

SUMMARY GUIDELINE

FATIGUE

INITIAL ASSESSMENT

- Exclude depression. Symptoms of this are: lethargy; tearfulness; anxiety; guilt; irritability; disturbed sleep patterns; lack of energy; poor appetite; poor concentration. If depression is suspected refer to guideline 7 on Depression and Other Psychological Morbidity

- Exclude anaemia. Ask about breathlessness, faintness, dizziness, tingling in fingers and toes. Check haemoglobin level. If low treat as local policy

- Exclude other physical or medical problems. If any are identified use appropriate guideline if available and/or refer to GP

WHAT TO DO

'SIMPLE' FATIGUE

- Help the woman plan her time each day to include short periods of rest. If possible ask a relative or friend to help
- Explain importance of exercise. Advise short daily walk when the woman feels she has most energy, which should then be followed by a short period of rest
- Check dietary intake adequate and stress need to eat regularly
- Where appropriate discuss social circumstances and lifestyle (e.g. young single mother). Referral to a health visitor may be arranged, if additional social support would be beneficial
- Encourage the woman to discuss any problems or worries she may have with the midwife and/or a close friend or family member
- It may be helpful if the woman keeps a diary of daily tasks to assess if fatigue is related to any particular activity or time of day and help her plan activity to include rest periods
- Review symptoms at subsequent visits
- Refer to GP if concerned about wellbeing at any time

REFERENCES

Atkinson L S, Baxley E G 1994 Postpartum fatigue. Am Fam Phys 50(1): 113–118
Bick D E, MacArthur C 1995 The extent, severity and effect of health problems after childbirth. Br J Midwif 3(1): 27–31
Brown S, Lumley J 1998 Maternal health after childbirth: results of an Australian population based survey. Br J Obstet Gynaecol 105: 156–161
Carty E M, Bradley C, Winslow W 1996 Women's perceptions of fatigue during pregnancy and postpartum: the impact of length of hospital stay. Clin Nurs Res 5(1): 67–80
Chen M K 1986 The epidemiology of self-perceived fatigue among adults. Prev Med 15: 74–81
Cox B, Blaxter M, Buckle A et al 1987 The health and lifestyles survey. Health Promotion Research Trust, London
David A, Pelosi A, McDonald E et al 1990 Tired, weak, or in need of rest: fatigue among general practice attenders. BMJ 301: 1199–1202
Fawcett J, York R 1986 Spouses' physical and psychological symptoms during pregnancy and the postpartum. Nurs Res 45: 144–148

Fulcher K Y, White P D 1997 Randomised controlled trial of graded exercise in patients with the chronic fatigue syndrome. BMJ 314: 1647–1652

Garcia J, Redshaw M, Fitzsimons B et al 1998 First class delivery. A national survey of women's views of maternity care. Audit Commission Publications, Abingdon, Oxford

Gardner D L 1991 Fatigue in postpartum women. Appl Nurs Res 4(2): 57–62

Gardner D L, Campbell B 1991 Assessing postpartum fatigue. Am J Matern Child Nurs 16(5): 264–266

Gjerdingen D K, Froberg D G 1991 The fourth stage of labor: the health of birth mothers and adoptive mothers at six-weeks postpartum. Fam Med 23(1): 29–35

Glazener C M A 1997 Sexual function after childbirth: women's experiences, persistent morbidity and lack of professional recognition. Br J Obstet Gynaecol 104: 330–335

Glazener C M, Abdalla M, Stoud P et al 1995 Postnatal maternal morbidity: extent, causes, prevention and treatment. Br J Obstet Gynaecol 102(4): 282–287

Gruis M 1977 Beyond maternity: postpartum concerns of mothers. Mat Child Nurs J May–June, pp 182–188

Hart L K, Freel M L, Milde F K 1990 Fatigue. Nurs Clin North Am 25(4): 967–976

Lee K A, Lentz M J, Taylor D L et al 1994 Fatigue as a response to environmental demands in women's lives. IMAGE: J Nurs Sch 26(2): 149–154

Loge J H, Ekeberg O, Kassa S 1998 Fatigue in the general Norwegian population: normative data and associations. J Psychomatic Res 45(1): 53–65

MacArthur C, Lewis M, Knox E G 1991 Health after childbirth. HMSO, London

Milligan R A, Pugh L C 1994 Fatigue during the childbearing period. Annu Rev Nurs Res 12: 33–49

Milligan R, Parks P, Lenz E 1990 An analysis of postpartum fatigue over the first three months of the postpartum period. In: Wang J, Simoni P, Nath C (eds) Vision of excellence: the decade of the nineties. West Virginia Nurses' Association Research Conference Group, Charlston, WV

Milligan R A, Flenniken P M, Pugh L C 1996 Positioning intervention to minimize fatigue in breastfeeding women. Appl Nurs Res 9(2): 67–70

North American Nursing Diagnosis Association (NANDA) 1990 Taxonomy I revisited—1990 with official nursing diagnoses. Mosby, St Louis

Oakley A 1992 The changing social context of pregnancy care. In: Chamberlain G, Zander L (eds) Pregnancy care in the 1990's. Parthenon, Carnforth

Parks P L, Lenz E R, Jenkins L S 1992 The role of social support and stressors for mothers and infants. Child Care Health Dev 18(3): 171

Paterson J A, Davis J, Gregory M et al 1994 A study of the effects of low haemoglobin on postnatal women. Midwifery 10: 77–86

Piper B F 1994 Fatigue: current bases for practice. In: Funk S G, Tornquist E M, Champagne M T et al (eds) Management of pain, fatigue and nausea. Macmillan, Basingstoke

Price J R, Couper J 2000 Cognitive behaviour therapy for chronic fatigue syndrome in adults. Cochrane Review 3. The Cochrane Library, Oxford

Pugh L C, Milligan R 1993 A framework for the study of childbearing fatigue. Adv Nurs Sci 15(4): 60–70

Rubin R 1975 Maternity nursing stops too soon. Am J Nurs 75: 1680–1684

Ruchala P L, Halstead L 1994 The postpartum experience of low-risk women: a time of adjustment and change. Mat Child Nurs J 22(3): 83–89

Saurel-Cubizolles M-J, Romito P, Lelong N et al 2000 Women's health after childbirth: a longitudinal study in France and Italy. Br J Obstet Gynaecol 107: 1201–1209

Smith-Hanrahan C, Deblois D 1995 Postpartum early discharge: impact on maternal fatigue and functional ability. Clin Nurs Res 4(1): 50–66

Tulman L, Fawcett J 1988 Return of functional ability after childbirth. Nurs Res 37(2): 77–81

Unterman R R, Posner N A, Williams K N 1990 Postpartum depressive disorders: changing trends. Birth 17: 131–137

Wambach K A 1998 Maternal fatigue in breastfeeding primiparae during the first nine weeks postpartum. J Hum Lactation 14(3): 219–229

Welford A T 1953 The psychologist's problem in measuring fatigue. In: Floyd W F, Welford A T (eds) Fatigue. Lewis, London, pp 183–191

Wessely S, Chalder T, Hirsch S et al 1996 Psychological symptoms, somatic symptoms and psychiatric disorder in chronic fatigue and chronic fatigue syndrome: a prospective study in the primary care setting. Am J Psychiat 153(8): 1050–1059

Wilkie G, Shapiro C M 1992 Sleep deprivation and the postnatal blues. J Psychosomatic Res 36(4): 309–316

9

Backache

INTRODUCTION

Women experience backache during pregnancy and following delivery. Most postpartum studies have not specified types of backache, but it is likely that most is simple backache. Nerve root pain (sciatica) and symphysis pubis pain, both of which can give rise to back pain, are also referred to in this guideline, although there are few studies on these symptoms among postnatal women.

SIMPLE BACKACHE

Definition

'Simple' backache is the term used to describe back pain which is musculo-skeletal in origin, mechanical in nature, varies with physical activity and time and can affect the lumbrosacral region, buttocks and thighs in a person who is generally well. The lower back is the most commonly reported site of pain (MacArthur et al 1991, Östgaard & Anderson 1992, Russell et al 1993, Turgut et al 1998).

Frequency of occurrence

Backache is very common during pregnancy, affecting 50% or more of all pregnant women to varying degrees (Berg et al 1988, Fast et al 1987, Östgaard et al 1991). It is thought to be triggered by hormonal factors and the increased weight of the gravid uterus (MacLennan et al 1986). Numerous observational studies have also shown backache to be common following childbirth, with a prevalence range of 20–50%. Garcia & Marchant (1993), in a postal questionnaire-based study of 90 women after delivery, found that 20% reported having backache at some time since their delivery. MacArthur et al (1991), in a study of 11 701 postnatal women questioned 1–9 years after the birth, found that 1634 (14%)

reported *new* backache (i.e. women without pregnancy or previous back-ache) which had started within 3 months of giving birth and lasted for longer than 6 weeks. Brown & Lumley (1998), in an Australian study of health among 1336 women at 6–7 months postpartum, found that back-ache occurring as a problem at some time since the birth was reported by 547 (44%) women.

Several studies have found that postpartum backache is often not tran-sient. Östgaard & Anderson (1991, 1992), in a Swedish cohort study, fol-lowed a representative sample of 817 women through pregnancy, at the end of which 67% reported back pain; at 12–18 month follow-up back pain prevalence was 37%. In a prospective observational study of a 20% sample (n = 1249) of women who delivered during one year in a region of Scotland, the women were given a questionnaire about health problems in hospital, then a postal questionnaire at 8 weeks postpartum, half receiving another at 12–18 months, to investigate subsequent problems. Backache was report-ed by 22% in hospital, by 24% between then and 8 weeks and by 20% after this (Glazener et al 1993). A postal questionnaire survey for the Audit Commission (Garcia et al 1998), of a sample of 2406 women throughout England and Wales at 4 months postpartum, asked about health problems as part of a wider study of maternity care. The women were asked to think back to 10 days, 1 month and 3 months and say which of a number of health problems they had at those times; 35% reported having had back-ache at 10 days, 27% at 1 month and 28% at 3 months. Among 1042 women delivering in a maternity unit in Boston, USA, 44% reported backache at 1–2 months postpartum (Breen et al 1994). At the 12–18 month follow-up, rates had not changed, with 49% experiencing back pain during the pre-ceding 3 months (Groves et al 1994). At the time of follow-up, backache was more common (66%) among the women who had reported backache in the 1–2 month questionnaire, compared with those who had not (21%). A recent longitudinal survey of the health of postpartum women in France (n = 589) and Italy (n = 697) followed up at 5 and 12 months, found a high prevalence of backache in each country at both times: 49% and 50% in France, and 47% and 65% in Italy. The Italian rates showed a surprising increase over the time (Saurel-Cubizolles et al 2000).

A few studies have examined the severity of postpartum back pain. Bick & MacArthur (1995) investigated the severity and effect of various post-natal morbidities, including backache, by postal questionnaire in a repre-sentative sample of 1278 women at 6–7 months postpartum. 582 women (46%) reported backache (new and recurrent) occurring within 3 months of birth and lasting for longer than 6 weeks, 49% of whom considered that it had affected their day to day activities. Mean severity of the backache, rated on a 100 mm visual analogue scale, was 39.4. Östgaard & Anderson (1992) found similar severity ratings of backache in their sample, with an average of 3.2 on a 10 cm visual analogue scale. Average pain severity before pregnancy in this same cohort (surveyed earlier using the same instruments) had been 0.99, and 4.4 during pregnancy (Östgaard & Anderson 1991). Serious postpartum backache was reported in this study by 7% of women at 12–18 months, similar to the Boston study (Groves et al 1994), where 8% reported severe back pain at this time.

Although backache is common following childbirth and can be persistent and affect daily life, studies have found medical consultation rates to be low (Bick & MacArthur 1995, Brown & Lumley 1998, MacArthur et al 1991). It should also be noted that general population-based epidemiological studies have found prevalence estimates of back pain to be high, 14–30% in studies asking about pain on that day and 30–40% in those asking about pain in the last month (Clinical Standards Advisory Group (CSAG) 1995). It is difficult to assess the extent of additional back pain that is attributable to childbirth.

Risk factors

A previous history of back pain is an important risk factor for postnatal backache and some studies have also found a relationship with physically demanding work. Östgaard & Anderson (1992), in the cohort study described earlier, found a significant association with back pain before pregnancy, sick leave for back pain during pregnancy, and physically heavy work (the researchers were not able to determine if the effect was from work before, during or after the pregnancy). Breen et al (1994), in the Boston study, also found a history of back pain to be predictive of postpartum back pain, but only if there had been back pain during pregnancy; those women who had back pain before, but not during, pregnancy were not at increased risk of postpartum back pain. Turgut et al (1998), in Turkey, followed 88 women who had suffered back pain during pregnancy to 6 months postpartum, and found that a history of pre-pregnancy back pain was a significant predictor of pain at 6 months, but found no relationship with heavy work before pregnancy. It is unclear, however, whether the women in this sample had suffered pregnancy back pain only in the current pregnancy or in any pregnancy; or whether the group comprised all women with pregnancy back pain during a defined time in the hospital or was subject to selection bias.

Breen et al (1994), in the Boston study, found younger maternal age and greater maternal weight to be predictors of postpartum backache and Brown & Lumley (1998) found an association with heavier infant birthweight. Glazener et al (1995) found a significant association with mode of delivery, with backache more likely after instrumental and caesarean deliveries, whilst in the study by Brown & Lumley (1998) there was proportionally more backache reported as a problem following these types of birth, but the difference was not statistically significant. MacArthur et al (1991) found an association with ethnic group, Asian women being much more likely to report backache as well as other musculoskeletal symptoms, although this may be due to cultural differences in the reporting of morbidity (MacArthur et al 1993).

The possibility of an association between epidural analgesia and postpartum backache has been investigated in several observational studies, some finding an association (Brown & Lumley 1998, MacArthur et al 1990, MacLeod et al 1995, Russell et al 1993), others not (Breen et al 1994, Macarthur et al 1995, Russell et al 1996). The first study to report on this relationship found that 18.9% of women reported *new* backache occurring within 3 months of delivery and lasting for over 6 weeks following epidural for pain relief, compared with 10.5% of those without. The suggested mechanism was through stressed postures in labour, affected by the hormone relaxin and exacerbated when morbidity and discomfort feedback are inhibited by epidural block. Russell et al (1993), in a similar study at St Thomas' Hospital, London among 612 primiparous women who received an epidural and 403 who did not, found a similar size epidural excess of new backache (17.8% vs 11.7%). In the Boston study (Breen et al 1994) of backache at 1–2 months postpartum, epidural use was associated neither with backache generally nor with new symptoms. The type of epidural given in this study centre, however, used a lower concentration of local anaesthetic together with an opiate, administered by a continuous infusion technique, which produces a less dense motor block and allows ambulation in many cases. The ability to move may reduce adverse effects of epidurals and is the subject of a current randomised controlled trial of mobile and non-mobile epidural techniques (COMET Study Group UK 2001, in press). In a small observational study from Canada (Macarthur et al 1995), 164 women who had an epidural and 165 who had not were interviewed at 1 and 7 days and 6 weeks after delivery. After excluding women who had had pregnancy backache, the only difference in new postpartum backache that reached statistical significance was on day 1 (52% epidural vs 39% non-epidural), although there was a two-fold epidural excess at 6 weeks (15% vs 7%). Among those followed up at 1 year, 10% had backache in the epidural and 14% in the non-epidural groups (Macarthur et al 1997).

A second study from St Thomas' Hospital, London (Russell et al 1996) compared women who requested an epidural, randomised to either a traditional (n = 157) or a mobile technique (n = 162), and a third group (n = 131) with no epidural, recruited by taking the next parity-matched delivery in the birth register. A postal questionnaire sent at 3 months postpartum found backache reported by 39% of the traditional group, 30% of the mobile group and 30.5% of the group with no epidural, and new backache was reported by 6.4%, 8.6% and 6.9% respectively. As in the study from Canada, since the differences were not statistically significant the authors concluded that women could be reassured that epidurals are not associated with postpartum backache. However, both studies were small with insufficient power to detect the size of difference found in the earlier studies.

All the above studies have been observational, and although they have used multivariate statistical analyses to confirm that the backache–epidural associations were independent of known confounders (since women who receive epidurals generally have less straightforward labours and deliveries), there remains the possibility that unknown differences might be producing the backache effect. A Cochrane systematic review (Howell 2000) which found 11 randomised controlled trials (RCTs) of epidural compared with other analgesia or with no analgesia for labour pain relief, found only one in which backache was an outcome measure. This showed no significant difference in backache at 6 months in women randomised to receive an epidural compared with pethidine, although only just over half of the women who consented to the trial actually took part and 40% of those randomised to pethidine actually had an epidural, making interpretation difficult and leaving the issue still unresolved (Loughnan et al 1997).

Management

There are no studies on the management of postpartum back pain. The evidence presented here, therefore, is based mainly on clinical guidelines prepared for the primary management of acute low back pain in the general population, first published by the Royal College of General Practitioners in 1996 and updated in 1999 (Waddell et al 1999). These guidelines build on a report of back pain by the CSAG (1995), who advise the UK government, and on the review which formed the basis of the US guidelines on back pain (Agency for Health Care Policy and Research (AHCPR) 1994). A subsequent systematic review on low back pain and sciatica in the BMJ Clinical Evidence series is also drawn on (van Tulder 1999). The RCGP guideline mainly refers to acute back pain but the Clinical Evidence review separately specifies evidence on chronic back pain, which is defined as persisting for 12 weeks or more.

The CSAG report stressed the importance of primary management of backache occurring within the first 6 weeks of onset, since any form of treatment once chronic pain is established has a lower chance of success (CSAG 1995). This is of particular relevance for postnatal management, since consultation rates for postpartum backache are low (Bick & MacArthur 1995, Brown & Lumley 1998, MacArthur et al 1991), highlighting the need to ask women specifically about symptoms to ensure prompt identification and management.

The guidelines present evidence relating to an assessment of the type of backache, including the role of psychological factors, and on management, the latter comprising symptomatic measures (drug therapy, bed rest, advice on staying active) and physical therapies (manipulation and back exercise).

Assessment

Assessment of the type of backache as simple or non-specific is first required to exclude possible serious spinal pathology and to distinguish nerve root pain or sciatica, for which management is slightly different (see later). There is now a great deal of evidence, with consistent findings from several prospective cohort studies, that psychosocial factors are particularly important in relation to chronic low back pain, that they influence a patient's response to treatment and rehabilitation and that they are important at a much earlier stage than previously believed (Waddell et al 1999).

Drugs, bedrest, advice to stay active

Management options for back pain have been extensively investigated with good quality evidence. In terms of *drug therapy*, analgesics (paracetamol, paracetamol–weak opioid compounds and NSAIDs) are all effective in reducing acute back pain. Comparisons between paracetamol and paracetamol–weak opioid compounds with NSAIDs are inconsistent, but the RCGP guidelines recommend paracetamol as first line drug therapy, followed by NSAIDs, then paracetamol–weak opioid compounds (such as co-dydramol or co-proxamol), probably because of side effects of the various preparations. RCTs examining a variety of muscle relaxants show that these are effective in reducing acute low back pain but there are side effects of drowsiness and dizziness and a risk of dependency (van Tulder 1999, Waddell et al 1999). For chronic back pain evidence suggests that analgesics and NSAIDs are both likely to be of benefit, but there is no evidence on muscle relaxants (van Tulder 1999).

The effectiveness of *bed rest* has been investigated in numerous RCTs which consistently show that this is not an effective treatment option, with adverse effects of prolonged bed rest such as joint stiffness and debilitation (van Tulder 1999, Waddell et al 1999). RCTs of *advice to stay active* are consistent in showing benefits of this in terms of faster rates of recovery, less pain, less sick leave and less chronic disability, compared with bed rest or with usual care. There are no studies, of an acceptable quality, of the effects of either bed rest or advice to stay active on chronic back pain.

Manipulation, back exercises

Physical therapies, both manipulation and back exercises, have been examined in a large number of RCTs, although many are of poor quality. For *manipulation* the RCGP guidelines (Waddell et al 1999) and the systematic review by van Tulder (1999) conclude that there are inconsistencies in the results. The RCGP report notes, however, that more of the trials report positive than negative results of manipulation in the short term improvement in pain and activity. Evidence on the effect of spinal manipulation on chronic back pain are conflicting. In relation to *back exercises*, RCTs show that it is doubtful that these produce clinically significant improvement in acute low back pain. For chronic pain, however, there is some evidence that exercise programmes can improve pain and functional levels, compared to conservative or a variety of inactive treatments (e.g. hot packs, TENS).

NERVE ROOT PAIN

Definition

Following the CSAG report (1995) and the RCGP guidelines (Waddell et al 1999), the term 'nerve root pain' is used here rather than 'sciatica', to emphasise specific clinical features which arise from nerve root irritation or entrapment, which is commonly caused by a disc prolapse. The pain generally arises from a single nerve root, and presents as relatively well localised, unilateral leg pain, often radiating into the foot or toes and associated with numbness or paraesthesia (CSAG 1995). The term sciatica is still used, however, by some back pain experts (van Tulder 1999, Vroomen et al 1999).

Frequency of occurrence

During pregnancy, symptoms of nerve root pain have been associated with the increased size of the uterus leading to backache and referred sciatica-like pain in the leg, and with prolapsed intervertebral disc, although this is rare (LaBan et al 1983). The only information on prolapsed discs in postnatal women has been presented in case reports (Ashkan et al 1998). The various studies of postpartum backache have not distinguished simple back pain and nerve root pain, so specific prevalences are unknown.

Management

Both the RCGP guidelines on acute back pain (Waddell et al 1999) and the Clinical Evidence review by van Tulder (1999) describe evidence specific to nerve root pain where this is available. The only real difference, however, is that although evidence on the effects of NSAIDs is inconsistent, the balance of it suggests that these are less effective for nerve root pain than for simple backache. Evidence for the other various therapies described for simple backache apply also to nerve root pain. A recent high quality RCT, specifically for patients with sciatica, of bed rest compared with watchful waiting found no evidence of effectiveness of bed rest (Vroomen et al 1999).

SYMPHYSIS PUBIS PAIN

Definition

Symphysis pubis pain can occur during pregnancy, in labour or following delivery. It is generally thought to be due to diastasis or separation of the pubic joint, as a result of hormonal or biomechanical factors affecting the laxity of the cartilage between the two pubic bones (Shepherd & Fry 1996). It is sometimes referred to as symphysis pubis diastasis (SPD) but it is not really known how often women have substantial widening without symptoms. Some widening of the pubic bones is considered to occur often during pregnancy, even up to as much as 10 mm, but it is suggested that symptoms are likely to occur if widening is greater than this (Lindsey et al 1988). Pain can present in the pubis, groins and lower back with referral to the thighs and legs. It can have a sudden or gradual onset, can be mild to severe and is exacerbated by walking and other weight bearing activities. A 'waddling' gait is typical and symphysial 'clicking' or grinding may occur (Fry et al 1997, Gamble et al 1986).

Frequency of occurrence and risk factors

The frequency of occurrence of symphysis pubis pain has been documented with considerable variation, one of the main UK textbooks for midwives quoting a range of case series over the years from 1 in 500 to 1 in 20 000 (Shepherd 1997). It is suggested that these variations are likely to be due to inconsistencies in diagnostic criteria and that since symphyseal separation may be mild and self limiting, underreporting is also likely to occur (Snow & Neubert 1997). In an American retrospective case note study of 5121 deliveries, nine cases occurred over a 2 year period, a rate of 1 in 569, five of these women having had antenatal symptoms (Snow & Neubert 1997). Another recent case series from one hospital in Wales, over a 21 month period, found that nine women were referred with symphysis pubis pain (Scriven et al 1995). During this time there had been 7350 births so, presuming there were no non-referred cases, the rate was around 1 in 800. In this study seven of the symptomatic women and 42 controls underwent ultrasound examination which showed that the median interpubic gap in the symptomatic women was 20 mm (range 10–35) compared with 4.8 mm (range 4.3–5.1) among the controls. These women were followed up to a median of 37 months, at which time four still had pubic pain. Persistent symptoms were not associated with a wider interpubic gap. In general it is considered that symptoms usually resolve by about 8 weeks postpartum (Lindsey et al 1988).

Since symphysis pubis pain is relatively uncommon, the only available information on risk factors is from case series. It is thought to be more frequent in multiparous women (Gamble et al 1986), with progressive weakening of the symphysis in successive deliveries leading to a higher risk of symptoms: eight of the nine cases in the series presented by Snow & Neubert (1997) were in multiparous women. A midwifery clinical review noted other risk factors as being related to delivery trauma, including precipitous labour, difficult instrumental delivery and cephalo-pelvic disproportion (Shepherd & Fry 1996).

Management

There are no trials evaluating treatment options for symphysis pubis pain and management of this was not included in the general population guidelines. Case series have suggested that conservative management during the acute phase is usually successful (Lindsey et al 1988). This includes bed rest until acute pain subsides (not recommended for simple backache) with hips adducted and the woman lying on her side, and pelvic support and analgesia (non-steroidal anti-inflammatory drugs such as ibuprofen) and the use of a pelvic binder or trochanteric belt (Shepherd 1997). Physiotherapy assessment is also thought to be beneficial (Fry et al 1997). Early intervention may assist recovery (Snow & Neubert 1997), therefore immediate referral to the GP is advised if the diagnosis is suspected by the midwife.

SUMMARY OF THE EVIDENCE USED IN THIS GUIDELINE

- Numerous large prospective studies have shown that backache is a common postpartum problem, occurring in 20–50% of women. Severe back pain occurs in under 10%. Backache after childbirth often persists; however, since prevalence is also high in the general population, the size of excess attributable to childbirth is difficult to assess.
- The most important risk factor for postpartum backache is a previous history of backache. Some studies have found a variety of other risk factors. Evidence on whether backache is associated with epidural analgesia is still inconclusive.
- Evidence from randomised controlled trials of the management of acute low back pain among the general population has shown that analgesics and advice to stay active are beneficial, but bed rest is ineffective. Psychological factors have an effect on treatment response. There is no specific evidence relating to postnatal management.
- The postnatal occurrence and management of nerve root pain has only been documented in case series. General population management is similar to simple backache.
- Symphysis pubis pain has been considered to be uncommon, but the only information available is from case series reports.

WHAT TO DO

INITIAL ASSESSMENT

The clinical history should take account of:

- The description of the symptom (for example, is it mostly in the back or does it refer to one or both legs, or is there any numbness or paraesthesia), and history and duration
- Any complicating psychosocial factors
- Symphysis pubis pain may present with or without back pain.

Following the RCGP guidelines (Waddell et al 1999), this will enable assessment of the backache as:

- Simple backache
- Nerve root pain (sciatica)
- Possible serious spinal pathology.

CONDITIONS WHICH REQUIRE IMMEDIATE REFERRAL TO GP

- Possible serious spinal pathology.
- Suspected nerve root pain (sciatica) radiating down one or both legs, especially when leg pain is severe.
- Symphysis pubis pain.

POSTPARTUM SIMPLE BACKACHE

- Analgesia (paracetamol as first line) should be taken on a regular basis to control pain.
- If paracetamol is not providing adequate pain relief, referral should be made to the GP for more powerful analgesia (NSAIDs or paracetamol–weak opioid compounds), ensuring advice is given about possible adverse side effects, such as constipation. For further advice, refer to 'Simple Pain Relief', Guideline 3.
- Advise the woman to continue with her normal activity as much as possible; since bed rest is ineffective and staying active leads to faster recovery.
- Depending on symptom severity, if there is no significant improvement after a week or two refer to the GP, since treatment within 6 weeks of onset is recommended (CSAG 1995).
- If the symptoms have not worsened, advise the woman to continue with normal activity and reduce the amount of analgesia she is taking.
- Psychological management, encouraging the woman to have a positive attitude, for example to activity and child care, is important. Back pain may be an indicator of psychological distress and depressive symptoms. (If this is suspected refer to guideline 7 on Depression and other psychological morbidity.)

Nerve root pain (sciatica)

- Initial management will follow the same principles as simple backache, but diagnosis and treatment by the GP is required.
- NSAIDs are proabably less effective than for simple backache.

Symphysis pubis pain

- Immediate referral to the GP should be made with symphysis pubis pain as early management, including analgesics (possibly NSAIDs) and physiotherapy referral, may be beneficial.
- Bed rest (lying on side) is likely to be necessary during the acute phase, which is of variable duration, and assistance with infant care during this phase will be required.
- Give explanation to woman, and her partner and family if appropriate.

General advice

- Reassure that backache is common after childbirth and that there are various successful management options available. Simple analgesia (paracetamol) and staying active (except for symphysis pubis pain) will help.

- The woman may benefit from practical advice: correct posture when handling, lifting and feeding the infant. The Association of Chartered Physiotherapists provides a simple leaflet which may be helpful, if available locally. Work through the literature with the woman to ensure that she understands it.

SUMMARY GUIDELINE

BACKACHE

INITIAL ASSESSMENT

- Ask about duration and description of problem
- Ask about any complicating psychosocial factors
- Ask about history of trauma

IMMEDIATE REFERRAL TO GP IS REQUIRED IF:

- Possible serious spinal pathology
- Suspected nerve root pain (sciatica); if pain radiating down one or both legs, especially if leg pain is severe
- Symphysis pubis pain
- Severe pain, especially affecting daily activities

WHAT TO DO

SIMPLE POSTPARTUM BACKACHE

- Analgesia (paracetamol as first line) should be taken on a regular basis
- If paracetamol is not satisfactory refer to GP for more powerful analgesia
- Advise to continue with normal activity, stay active and not to take bed rest
- If no significant improvement, refer to GP as treatment within 6 weeks of onset is recommended
- Psychological management should include the encouragement of a positive attitude to activity and child care

NERVE ROOT PAIN (SCIATICA)

- Initial management as for simple backache, but diagnosis and treatment by GP is required
- NSAIDs are probably less effective than for simple backache

SYMPHYSIS PUBIS PAIN

- GP referral should be made, as stronger analgesia and physiotherapy referral may be appropriate
- Bed rest is necessary during the acute phase, which is of variable duration
- Give explanation to woman, her partner and family, if appropriate

GENERAL ADVICE

- Reassure that backache is common after childbirth and there are various successful management options available. It will improve with simple analgesia and normal activity which will reduce the risk of problem becoming chronic
- Give the woman a copy of the leaflet from The Association of Chartered Physiotherapists (if available)
- Advise on correct posture when handling, lifting and feeding the infant

REFERENCES

AHCPR 1994 Management guidelines for acute low back pain. Agency for Health Care Policy and Research, US Department of Health and Human Service, Rockville, MD

Ashkan K, Casey A T H, Powell M et al 1998 Back pain during pregnancy and after childbirth: an unusual cause not to miss. J R Soc Med 91: 88–90

Berg G, Hammar M, Moller-Nielsen J et al 1988 Low back pain during pregnancy. Obstet Gynecol 71(1): 71–75

Bick D, MacArthur C 1995 The extent, severity and effect of health problems after childbirth. Br J Midwif 3(1): 27–31

Breen T W, Ransil B J, Groves P A et al 1994 Factors associated with back pain after childbirth. Anesthesiology 81(1): 29–34

Brown S, Lumley J 1998 Maternal health after childbirth: results of an Australian population based survey. Br J Obstet Gynaecol 105: 156–161

Clinical Standards Advisory Group 1995 Back pain. Chaired by Professor Michael Rosen. HMSO, London

COMET Study Group UK The effect of low dose 'mobile' compared with traditional epidural techniques on mode of delivery: a randomised controlled trial. Lancet in press

Fast A, Shapiro D, Ducommun E J et al 1987 Low back pain during pregnancy. Spine 12: 368–371

Fry D, Hay-Smith J, Hough J et al 1997 National clinical guideline for the care of women with symphysis pubis dysfunction. Midwives 110(1314): 172–173

Gamble J G, Simmons S C, Freedman M 1986 The symphysis pubis. Anatomic and pathologic considerations. Clin Orthop 203: 261–272

Garcia J, Marchant S 1993 Back to normal? Postpartum health and illness. In: Robinson S, Tickner V (eds) Research and the midwife. Conference proceedings 1992. University of Manchester

Garcia J, Redshaw M, Fitzsimons B et al 1998 First class delivery. A national survey of women's views of maternity care. Audit Commission Publications, Abingdon, Oxford

Glazener C, Abdalla M, Russell I et al 1993 Postnatal care: a survey of patients' experiences. Br J Midwif 1(2): 67–74

Glazener C, Abdalla M, Stoud P et al 1995 Postnatal maternal morbidity: extent, causes, prevention and treatment. Br J Obstet Gynaecol 102(4): 282–287

Groves P A, Breen T W, Ransil B J et al 1994 Natural history of post partum back pain and its relationship with epidural anesthesia. Anesthesiology 81(3A): A1167

Howell C J 2000 Epidural versus non-epidural analgesia in pain relief in labour. Cochrane Review 3. The Cochrane Library, Oxford

LaBan M M, Perrin J C S, Latimer F R 1983 Pregnancy and the herniated lumbar disc. Arch Phys Med Rehabil 64: 319–321

Lindsey R W, Leggon R E, Wright D G et al 1988 Separation of the symphysis pubis in association with childbearing. J Bone Joint Surg 70-A(2): 289–292

Loughnan B A, Carli F, Romney M et al 1997 The influence of epidural analgesia on the development of new backache in primiparous women: report of a randomised controlled trial. Int J Obstet Anaes 6: 203–204

Macarthur A, MacArthur C, Weeks S K 1995 Epidural anaesthesia and low back pain after delivery: a prospective cohort study. BMJ 311: 1336–1339

Macarthur A J, MacArthur C, Weeks S K 1997 Is epidural anesthesia in labor associated with chronic low back pain? A prospective cohort study. Anesth Analg 85: 1066–1070

MacArthur C, Lewis M, Knox E G et al 1990 Epidural anaesthesia and long term backache after childbirth. BMJ 301: 9–12

MacArthur C, Lewis M, Knox E G 1991 Health after childbirth. HMSO, London

MacArthur C, Lewis M, Knox E G 1993 Comparison of long-term health problems following childbirth in Asian and Caucasian women. Br J Gen Pract 42: 519–522

MacLennan A H, Nicholson R, Green R C et al 1986 Serum relaxin and pelvic pain of pregnancy. Lancet ii: 243–245

MacLeod J, Macintyre C, McClure J H et al 1995 Backache and epidural analgesia. Int J Obstet Anesth 4: 21–25

Östgaard H C, Anderson G B J 1991 Previous back pain and risk of developing back pain in a future pregnancy. Spine 16(4): 432–436

Östgaard H C, Anderson G B J 1992 Postpartum low-back pain. Spine 17: 53–55

Östgaard H C, Anderson G B J, Karlsson K 1991 Prevalence of back pain in pregnancy. Spine 16: 549–552

Russell R, Groves P, Taub N et al 1993 Assessing long term backache after childbirth. BMJ 306: 1299–1303

Russell R, Dundas R, Raynolds F 1996 Long term backache after childbirth: prospective search for causative factors. BMJ 312: 1384–1388

Saurel-Cubizolles M-J, Romito P, Lelong N et al 2000 Women's health after childbirth: a longitudinal study in France and Italy. Br J Obstet Gynaecol 107: 1202–1209

Scriven M W, Jones D A, McKnight L 1995 The importance of pubic pain following childbirth: a clinical and ultrasonographic study of diastasis of the pubic symphysis. J R Soc Med 88: 28–30

Shepherd J 1997 Helping women cope with pregnancy changes. In: Sweet B (ed) Mayes' midwifery. A textbook for midwives. Baillière Tindall, London, ch 20

Shepherd J, Fry D 1996 Symphysis pubis pain. Midwives 109(1302): 199–201

Snow R E, Neubert A G 1997 Peripartum pubic symphysis separation: a case series and review of the literature. Obstet Gynecol Surv 52(7): 438–443

Turgut F, Turgut M, Çetinsahin M 1998 A prospective study of persistent back pain after pregnancy. Eur J Obst Gynecol Reprod Biol 80: 45–48

van Tulder M 1999 Low back pain and sciatica. In: Clinical evidence. British Medical Journal Publications 2: 406–422

Vroomen P C A J, de Krom M C T F M, Wilmink J T et al 1999 Lack of effectiveness of bed rest for sciatica. N Engl J Med 340(6): 418–423

Waddell G, McIntosh A, Hutchinson A et al 1999 Low back pain evidence review. Royal College of General Practitioners, London

10

Headache

INTRODUCTION

The two types of headache most commonly reported among the general population are tension headache and migraine, both of which are more frequent among women, possibly related to hormonal factors (Rasmussen 1993). Whether these types of headache are more common among postpartum than non-postpartum women is not known, since there are no comparative studies. There is some information, however, about headaches in the postnatal period from studies of health problems in postpartum populations. In addition, there are some conditions which are more common among postnatal women and which can present with, or result in, headaches. These are: post-dural puncture headaches following spinal or epidural anaesthesia; headache associated with postpartum hypertension, pre-eclampsia or eclampsia; and sub-arachnoid haemorrhage. All of these are reviewed in this guideline.

Definition

According to the International Headache Society's diagnostic criteria, a tension-type headache is usually bilateral and includes pressing or tightening feelings, is of mild or moderate intensity, has no nausea or vomiting, and is not aggravated by routine physical activity. Phonophobia or photophobia are possible, but not both. A migraine headache tends to be unilateral and pulsating, of moderate to severe intensity, is aggravated by routine physical activity and is accompanied by at least two symptoms of nausea, vomiting, photophobia and phonophobia (International Headache Society 1988). It is likely that these are the types of headaches experienced by postpartum women but most studies do not specify type.

181

POSTPARTUM HEADACHE

Frequency of occurrence and risk factors

Studies that have examined the occurrence of headaches early after child-birth suggest that these are experienced by 20–40% of women on 1 or more days during the first week (Grove 1973, Pitt 1973, Stein 1981, Stein et al 1984). Garcia & Marchant (1993), in an observational study of postnatal health at 8 weeks among 90 women, found that 23% had experienced headaches at some time since the birth. Longer term studies in postpartum populations have also found frequent headaches to be common. In one large observational study of a variety of health problems after childbirth, 419 (4%) of 11 701 women reported frequent headaches which had begun for the first time within 3 months of the delivery and lasted for over 6 weeks, and a further 5% reported similar frequent headaches which they had also had sometime before. The corresponding proportions reporting migraine were 1% and 6%, indicating that migraine was less likely to be a *new* postpartum problem (MacArthur et al 1991). Glazener et al (1995), in a prospective observational study, examined maternal postnatal morbidity in over 1200 women, who comprised a 20% random sample of deliveries in the Grampian region of Scotland between June 1990 and May 1991. All women were given a questionnaire whilst on the postnatal ward, a postal questionnaire at 8 weeks, and half were sent another questionnaire 12–18 months after the birth. Headaches of any duration, including new and recurrent symptoms, were reported by 14% of women whilst in hospital, by 22% between then and 8 weeks and by 15% after this.

A recent longitudinal survey of Italian and French women's health after childbirth found that headache prevalence had increased at 12 months postpartum compared with at 5 months: 45% of Italian women reported headaches at 12 months compared with 22% at 5 months, 38% of French women had headaches at 12 months compared with 21% at 5 months (Saurel-Cubizolles et al 2000).

An additional finding of MacArthur et al (1991) was that headaches occurring with musculoskeletal symptoms often starting during the first postnatal week were more likely to occur in women who had epidural analgesia for pain relief. Frequent headaches or migraine without muscu-loskeletal symptoms were associated with younger age, multiparity and lower social class, and not with epidural analgesia, and were probably related more to factors within the social environment than to the delivery. Headaches in the first postpartum week were found to be associated with psychological morbidity by Stein et al (1984). In this study, the occurrence of headache was documented daily among 71 women by them completing a self-rating questionnaire, which also included questions on the presence of tension, depression and feelings of weepiness. Women who developed a headache on at least 1 day were more depressed and had more tension than those who did not. Details of the self-rating schedule were not described, thus its validity cannot be assessed.

Management

Studies of headache after hospital discharge were all investigating post-natal health more generally, and relied on self-reports of headaches, without obtaining detailed classificatory information necessary to distinguish different types of headache, as in the International Headache Society classification. It is likely, however, that most postpartum headaches are tension headaches, the next most common being migraine, most of which will be reported by women who have a previous history of this. The main role of the midwife is to assess the headache in order to refer those that are due to other causes. The management of tension headaches and migraine is the same as for general population groups (Barrett 1996), taking care that any analgesia is appropriate for breastfeeding mothers.

POST-DURAL PUNCTURE HEADACHE

Definition

A post-dural puncture headache (PDPH) may occur following the administration of an epidural or spinal needle for pain relief in labour or for caesarean section. In the case of spinal anaesthesia the dura is punctured deliberately, whilst an accidental dural puncture occurs occasionally during the insertion of the epidural needle. The diagnosis of an accidental dural puncture is usually made by the anaesthetist during insertion of the epidural, when cerebrospinal fluid (CSF) is observed, but some cases are diagnosed retrospectively following the onset of headache in the puerperium.

Headache after dural puncture results from a loss of CSF, with subsequent traction on the meninges, and has several typical presenting characteristics. The most significant is its postural nature; the headache gets dramatically worse when the patient moves from the supine to the upright position, and conversely is markedly diminished or relieved totally when the patient is lying down (Katz & Aidinis 1980). The associated symptoms of neck stiffness, visual disturbances, vomiting and auditory symptoms may also be reported, but are more common with severe PDPH (Lybecker et al 1995).

Frequency of occurrence and risk factors

The incidence of accidental dural puncture during epidural is now between about 0.5% and 1%, although it had been higher than this when epidural was first used in routine obstetric practice (Stride & Cooper 1993). Where this type of puncture does occur, however, the relatively large diameter of the epidural needle means that loss of CSF is likely and the incidence of

PDPH is high. This high incidence is also attributed to bearing down in the second stage of labour, which may exacerbate CSF leakage; to decreased intra-abdominal pressure following delivery, which causes the epidural veins to collapse; and to rapid loss of fluid from blood loss, diuresis and lactation (Gutsche 1990). In a case note analysis of 20 years of women with accidental puncture in one maternity unit, the incidence of typical PDPH was 86% (Stride & Cooper 1993). The majority of the women (69%) in this series developed their headache within the first 2 days of delivery, although it sometimes did not appear until at least 6 days after (Stride & Cooper 1993). Most PDPHs are of relatively short duration, lasting for several days (Crawford 1972). In the study described earlier, however, of health problems after childbirth 74 of the 11 701 women, were recorded as having an accidental dural puncture and 23% of these reported frequent headaches or migraine lasting for longer than 6 weeks. Information on whether these headaches were of a postural nature was not obtained, although some women also reported neckache or visual or auditory disturbances (MacArthur et al 1993).

Much smaller diameter needles are used for spinal than for epidural analgesia, so that although a spinal always punctures the dura, with current types of spinal needles (see below) similar proportions of PDPHs occur after each procedure. Spinal anaesthesia has been used for a variety of surgical and investigative interventions for 100 years or so, but the early incidence of PDPH was high. In a classic study from the USA of a general series of 10 098 spinals, it was noted that obstetric patients had the highest headache rates (Vandam & Dripps 1956). In 1979 Crawford reported a PDPH rate of 16% in an obstetric unit that was a specialist centre for regional blocks (Crawford 1979). Spinal needles of smaller diameter and designs that spread rather than cut the dural fibres have since become popular. A general population based meta-analysis, which found rates of all headaches ranging from 1% to almost 30%, and rates of severe headaches from 0 to 12%, concluded that smaller and non-cutting needles were associated with the lowest rates (Halpern & Preston 1994). A randomised controlled trial of spinal anaesthesia for caesarean section compared a 25 gauge diamond tipped needle with a 24 gauge non-cutting Sprotte needle (Cesarini et al 1990). The trial planned to recruit 100 women to each group but was stopped at 55, when a PDPH rate of 14.5% was shown in the former group, compared with none in the Sprotte group. Other obstetric studies comparing different needles have had similar findings (e.g. Shutt et al 1992). Most maternity units now report incidence rates of severe headaches requiring blood patch of about 1% or less (Hopkinson et al 1997, Madej et al 1993). Mild headaches have been documented in up to 10% (Hopkinson et al 1997), but the extent to which these might be attributed to the spinal is not known since, as described earlier, headaches in the first few days after birth are generally quite common.

Management

Since many women are now discharged from hospital before a PDPH is likely to develop, it is important that the midwife is able to identify this type of headache (Cooper 1999). For PDPH referral must be made to the obstetric anaesthetist or the GP, according to local policy. In the case of a known accidental dural puncture the anaesthetist may have already instituted prophylactic measures or begun treatment if symptoms were severe.

A clinical review of the treatment of PDPH in the general population notes that conservative treatment of PDPH is recommended in the first instance, which includes simple analgesics (e.g. paracetamol), bed rest and hydration. Bed rest seems to alleviate symptoms, although this has not been found to be effective in preventing a headache occurring (McSwiney & Phillips 1995). There have been no systematic reviews, however, of these commonly used treatments in either obstetric or general populations. An evaluation of the literature (including clinical studies, letters, abstracts and case reports) on the pharmacological management of PDPH in general populations concluded that intravenous and oral caffeine are effective treatments, and anyway non-invasive, but that more clinical studies are required to properly evaluate other pharmacotherapies. In the meantime the authors suggest that therapy be guided by clinical judgement (Choi et al 1996).

Epidural blood patch is now considered by many obstetric anaesthetists to be an effective treatment for severe PDPH after accidental puncture or spinal anaesthesia. This involves injecting 10–20 ml of the woman's blood into the epidural space around the site of the dural puncture; the blood coagulates and seals the leak of CSF. A second blood patch is sometimes given in the event of failure. A success rate of over 90% has been reported in some observational studies, although others report permanent symptom relief in about two thirds of cases (Stride & Cooper 1993, Taivainen et al 1993), and the technique has never been subject to systematic review (Sudlow & Warlow 2000). There is controversy about the use of blood patching as a prophylactic measure where accidental dural puncture is known to have occurred (Cooper 1999). Berger et al (1998), in a survey of the management of accidental dural puncture during labour in 36 centres in North America, found that almost half used prophylactic blood patching.

HYPERTENSIVE DISORDERS

Much has been written on the hypertensive disorders of pregnancy and there are various differing definitions. It is included in this guideline because headache can be one of its manifestations and because these disorders can occur in the postpartum period.

Hypertension

Pregnancy induced hypertension (PIH) was defined in a clinical review of the hypertensive disorders of pregnancy as the recording of a blood pressure of 140/90 mmHg or more on two occasions 4 or more hours apart after the twentieth week of pregnancy, in a previously normotensive woman (Broughton Pipkin 1995). Some postnatal women may have chronic or essential hypertension, defined as a blood pressure recording greater than 140/90 mmHg, present prior to pregnancy or before 20 weeks' gestation (Magee et al 1999).

Frequency of occurrence

Around 5–10% of pregnant women will develop PIH (Broughton Pipkin 1995, Magee et al 1999). There are few studies, however, that have examined the prevalence of hypertension in the postpartum period. Walters et al (1986) measured the blood pressure of 136 previously normotensive women in the morning and afternoon for 5 days following normal delivery. Both systolic and diastolic blood pressure rose for the first 4 days, leading the authors to conclude that a rise in blood pressure during this period seems to represent a general phenomenon. Other studies have examined the postnatal duration of hypertension among women who have already presented with PIH or pre-eclampsia. Ferrazzani et al (1994) studied 269 women with PIH (n = 159) or pre-eclampsia (n = 110) and monitored their postpartum blood pressure daily after delivery until a diastolic blood pressure of ≤110 mmHg was reached. The time taken for this ranged from 0 to 10 days among the PIH women and from 0 to 23 days among those with pre-eclampsia. How long it took for women to become normotensive (diastolic ≤80 mmHg), however, was not reported.

In addition to headache, other symptoms that sometimes accompany a rise in blood pressure include photophobia, visual disturbances, vomiting or epigastric discomfort, although these are less likely to occur in less severe cases.

Management

A recent review in the British Medical Journal of the management of hypertension in pregnancy identified three randomised controlled trials, involving a total of 136 women, that have examined this during the first 48 hours after delivery (Magee et al 1999). Based on this limited evidence the review concluded that, pending further studies, women should continue taking hypertensive medication after delivery, and clinicians should continue to prescribe treatments they are familiar with. Hypertensive women will require regular monitoring of their blood pressure and urinalysis in order that referral to the GP or obstetrician could be made if indicated. How frequent the monitoring should be will be based on discussion with the woman's medical advisors.

Postpartum pre-eclampsia and eclampsia

Pre-eclampsia is considered to occur when pregnancy induced hypertension is associated with significant proteinurea (300 mg/l in 24h) (Davey & MacGillivray 1988). The precise relationship between PIH and pre-eclampsia, however, is still unclear. The most common definition of *eclampsia* is convulsions, plus the usual signs and symptoms of pre-eclampsia, where other causes of convulsion have been excluded (Douglas & Redman 1994).

Frequency of occurrence

Douglas & Redman (1994) undertook a prospective survey of all hospitals with a consultant obstetric unit, as well as questionnaires to GPs, to document the incidence of eclampsia in the United Kingdom in 1992. The precise definition of eclampsia used in the survey was the occurrence of convulsions during pregnancy, labour or within 10 postpartum days, together with at least two of the following within 24 hours of the convulsion: hypertension, proteinuria, thrombocytopenia or raised plasma aspartate transaminase concentration. The number of cases identified was 383, an incidence of 4.9 per 10 000 maternities, and 1 in 50 of the women died. Most (85%) women had been seen by a doctor or midwife in the preceding week; 43% of these had not had hypertension with proteinuria, and some (11%) had had neither of these signs. Antecedent symptoms had been experienced by 59% of the eclamptic women: 50% had headaches, 19% visual disturbances and 19% epigastric pain. Among all the women with eclampsia, 44% were found to occur in the postpartum period. The proportion of postpartum cases occurring without hypertension, proteinuria or antecedent symptoms is not given, but expert opinion suggests that it is unlikely to be different from the overall pattern.

Lubarsky et al (1994) undertook a 15 year (1977–1992) case note review in one unit in the USA to investigate *late* postpartum eclampsia—convulsions which occurred between 48 hours and 4 weeks postpartum. During this period 112 500 women delivered and there was a total of 334 cases of eclampsia. Among these, 97 (29%) occurred postpartum, 54 of which were classed as late postpartum, occurring as long as 23 days after delivery, although most occurred much earlier than this. Of the 54 women with late postpartum eclampsia, 45 (83%) had prodromal symptoms: 38 (70%) reported severe headache and 17 (31%) visual disturbances, with some women reporting both symptoms. The duration of symptoms prior to convulsion was between 2 and 72 hours. The authors noted that the subjective signs and symptoms of severe and persistent occipital headache, photophobia, blurred vision or scotomata and epigastric pain can serve as clinical warning before the onset of convulsions. The majority of late post-partum convulsions in this study occurred after hospital discharge.

Atterbury et al (1998), in a retrospective case control study, identified 57 women from 32 762 in one unit who were subsequently readmitted with severe pre-eclampsia or eclampsia at a rate of 1.7 per 1000 maternities. Four women were excluded because of incomplete case notes and the remaining 53 (32 with pre-eclampsia and 21 with eclampsia) were matched two-to-one with 106 women who had intrapartum severe pre-eclampsia or eclampsia. Detailed information on symptoms, physical findings and laboratory assays were obtained. The case control comparison showed that headache, visual disturbances, nausea and vomiting and malaise were reported significantly more by postpartum women on readmission, than by controls during labour or in the immediate postpartum period. The occurrence of oedema and epigastric pain did not vary between cases and controls. In postpartum women headaches were positively correlated with systolic, diastolic and mean arterial blood pressure, but this relationship was not found in the control group. Women readmitted with symptoms were more likely to develop seizures than women in the control group.

Management

Although routine antenatal screening measures may enable the detection of women at risk of pre-eclampsia and eclampsia, it is important to note, as shown above, that eclamptic seizures can occur without antenatal indicators and can occur after hospital postnatal discharge. Eclampsia can occur unheralded by signs and possibly even by symptoms, and certainly with only short duration ones. Women may have an eclamptic fit despite previously having a relatively low diastolic blood pressure (Douglas & Redman 1994). Community midwives must therefore be alert to all possible warning signs and symptoms. Where a woman has hypertension and complains of a headache in the postpartum period and there are symptoms of pre-eclampsia, such as epigastric discomfort, visual disturbance, nausea or vomiting, an urgent referral should be made to the GP.

Duley et al (2000) undertook a Cochrane systematic review of 10 trials, including over 3000 antenatal and postnatal women, of anticonvulsant therapies for pre-eclampsia. This showed that use of anticonvulsants compared with no anticonvulsants was associated with a reduced risk of eclampsia (RR 0.33, 95% CI 0.11–1.02); and that magnesium sulphate appeared to be more effective than phenytoin at reducing the risk of eclampsia (RR 0.05, 95% CI 0.00–0.84), but there was an increased risk of caesarean section (RR 1.21, 95% CI 1.05–1.41). Studies comparing magnesium sulphate with diazepam were too small to enable reliable conclusions. The reviewers concluded that there was insufficient evidence to establish the benefit and hazards of anticonvulsants for women with pre-eclampsia. However, if an anticonvulsant is used, magnesium sulphate appears to be the best choice.

Two Cochrane systematic reviews of the treatment for eclampsia (Duley & Henderson-Smart 2000a, 2000b) both examining magnesium sulphate, one compared with diazepam and the other compared with phenytoin, have concluded that magnesium sulphate appears to be substantially more effective in reducing the recurrence of convulsions than each of the other treatments for eclampsia (RR for diazepam 0.45, 95% CI 0.35–0.58; RR for phenytoin 0.30, 95% CI 0.20–0.46).

SUB-ARACHNOID HAEMORRHAGE (SAH)

Definition

A sub-arachnoid haemorrhage is a bleed into the sub-arachnoid space. It often presents with a violent and unusual headache, often described as thunderclap. Case reports of non-puerperal cases have described presenting symptoms as including sudden severe headache and vomiting (Wasserberg & Barlow 1997).

Frequency of occurrence and risk factors

In the most recent triennial report on confidential enquiries into maternal deaths in the UK 1994–1996 (Department of Health 1998) no deaths were attributed to SAH; however two postpartum deaths were attributed to SAH in the report for the previous two years (Department of Health 1996). SAH, although extremely rare, is associated with poor outcome, with a general population-based case fatality rate of around 40% (van Gijn 1997). A literature review of cerebrovascular pathology during pregnancy and postpartum found a mean incidence of SAH of 20 per 100 000 deliveries. This is about five times greater than outside parturition, although the reviewers noted methodological weaknesses in some of the studies (Lamy et al 1996). It is suggested that the haemodynamic, hormonal or other physiological changes of pregnancy may play a role in increasing the likelihood of aneurysmal rupture (Lamy et al 1996).

A systematic review of risk factors for SAH in the general population was carried out, which included nine longitudinal studies and 11 case control studies (Teunissen et al 1996). Smoking, hypertension and alcohol were found to be the most significant risk factors. No studies were identified, however, that had examined risk factors for SAH in postpartum populations, although among females generally neither oral contraceptive use nor HRT have shown any association.

Management

With such a high case fatality rate, early referral of SAH to a specialist centre is essential. Diagnosis is usually confirmed using CT scan and lumbar puncture (Sztark et al 1996). On average GPs will only encounter a patient with an SAH every 8 years (Linn et al 1996). It is likely that most midwives will never see a case in a postpartum woman, although patients presenting with a sudden and violent or severe headache should be taken seriously. The midwife should refer immediately to the GP, who is likely to refer to a specialist neurological centre.

SUMMARY OF THE EVIDENCE USED IN THIS GUIDELINE

- Large observational studies have found that headaches are relatively common after childbirth, although there are no comparative studies of postpartum and non-postpartum women.
- Observational studies have shown that PDPH can occur after spinal anaesthesia and trials have shown lower rates with smaller diameter and non-cutting needles.
- Although accidental puncture during epidural is uncommon, case series have shown that the incidence of PDPH after this is very high.
- Further studies, including randomised controlled trials, are required to assess the long term effectiveness of treatments commonly used to *manage* symptoms of PDPH following epidural or spinal anaesthesia.
- Few studies have investigated the prevalence of *postpartum* hypertensive disorders.
- Only three small trials, included in one review paper, have addressed the management of postpartum hypertension.
- Various types of descriptive studies of eclampsia have shown that this can be unheralded by signs and there may be a very short duration of symptoms or even an absence prior to convulsion; and that 29–44% of all cases of eclampsia occur in the postnatal period.
- Sub-arachnoid haemorrhage presenting with a sudden violent headache is extremely rare, but often fatal.

WHAT TO DO

INITIAL ASSESSMENT

This is in order to exclude possible diagnoses other than tension headache or migraine.

- Ask about the onset of the headache, the location and duration. Has the woman suffered any trauma to the head?
- If the woman had epidural/spinal analgesia, is the headache relieved by lying down?
- Ask about other conditions that produce, exacerbate or relieve the headache.
- Check essential or pregnancy related hypertension. Obtain baseline recording of blood pressure if appropriate (if hypertensive see section below).
- What degree of incapacity does the headache cause, i.e. can the woman carry out normal activities, do the headaches interfere with or prevent sleep?

THE SYMPTOMS LISTED BELOW ARE NOT TYPICAL AND IMMEDIATE GP REFERRAL IS REQUIRED

- Complaints of violent and sudden onset ('thunderclap') headache possibly with vomiting.
- Generalised headache where there is intense pain in the back of the neck or signs of fever.
- Headache associated with trauma.
- Progressively worsening headache.
- BP of 160/100 or higher.
- Headache with other symptoms of pre-eclampsia.

SYMPTOMS SUGGESTIVE OF POSTPARTUM 'SIMPLE HEADACHE' (TENSION HEADACHE OR MIGRAINE)

- If known migraine sufferer continue with usual medication.
- Simple analgesia can be advised—try paracetamol. If analgesia is insufficient or further assessment required, refer to GP.
- If the woman has learnt relaxation techniques during the antenatal period she should be encouraged to continue these to relieve tension. If not, give advice on these.
- Discuss changes in child care. Explore ways to ensure sufficient sleep, e.g. relative/friend may care for the baby for a period during the day when the mother can rest.
- Attempt to identify with the woman any factors which may trigger the headache, and ways in which these can be avoided.
- Reassure the woman that this type of headache is common and is generally no major cause for concern.

SYMPTOMS SUGGESTIVE OF PDPH

- Where PDPH is suspected referral should be made to the relevant anaesthetic department at the hospital where the woman delivered or the GP. Some women may require hospital admission for assessment and treatment (blood patch).

- If the headache is severe, the woman should be encouraged to lie down and rest, to alleviate symptoms since the headache is usually postural. Bed rest will not *prevent* headaches.

- It is common practice to check and record blood pressure/temperature/pulse to obtain baseline.

- Where symptoms are moderate, include simple analgesia advice (see 'Simple Pain Relief' section, Guideline 3) in addition to reassurance.

- Hydration might help so check that fluid intake is adequate.

- Caffeine might help.

- Advise woman about possible diagnosis and that treatment is available.

- Ensure woman has available support to help her care for her infant and herself whilst she is experiencing the headaches.

- Visit as required to assess progress.

HEADACHE ASSOCIATED WITH HYPERTENSIVE DISORDERS

- Where a woman complains of headache in the postpartum period, has hypertension and there are other symptoms of pre-eclampsia, such as epigastric discomfort, visual disturbance, nausea or vomiting, an urgent referral should be made to the GP.

- Moderate hypertension in an otherwise well woman is fine. For these women expert opinion suggests that an upper limit of 160/100 can generally be taken as an appropriate action threshold in order to pick up those who are likely to go higher (i.e. ≥170/100, which can exceed limits of cerebral auto-regulation and therefore predispose to stroke). For women with blood pressure of 160/100 mmHg or higher, urgent referral should be made to the GP.

- If the woman complains of severe headache and has a history of hypertension in pregnancy, GP referral should be made.

- Known essential hypertension is less worrying than a history of hypertension in pregnancy; continue management as medical instructions, ensure that the woman has appropriate follow-up. Immediate GP referral should be made if the woman has signs or symptoms of pre-eclampsia (see above).

- If hypertension is uncomplicated the woman should be reassured and simple analgesia given for the headache.

- In all the above cases review the woman the following day.

- Discuss any concerns about hypertensive disorders in a woman with her GP at any time if indicated.

SUMMARY GUIDELINE

HEADACHE

INITIAL ASSESSMENT

To exclude diagnoses other than tension headache/migraine:

- Ask about onset, location and duration of headache. History of trauma?
- Did the woman have epidural/spinal analgesia, and is headache postural? (Possible PDPH)
- Are there other conditions which produce, exacerbate or relieve the headache?
- Is there a history of hypertension?
- What degree of incapacity does the headache produce?

IMMEDIATE REFERRAL TO GP IS REQUIRED IF:

- Severe and sudden onset of 'thunderclap' headache
- Headache associated with neck stiffness, pyrexia, signs of fever
- Headache associated with trauma
- Symptoms of pre-eclampsia (hypertension, headache, epigastric pain, visual disturbances, nausea or vomiting)
- BP ≥160/100 mmHg

WHAT TO DO

POSTPARTUM 'SIMPLE' HEADACHE

- If known migraine sufferer, continue with usual medication
- Mild analgesia (paracetamol) can be advised. If analgesia insufficient refer to GP
- Advise on relaxation
- Discuss child care and sleep—ways to have a rest during the day
- Attempt to identify factors which trigger headache
- Reassure that this type of headache is common and is generally no cause for concern

SYMPTOMS OF PDPH

- Contact anaesthetic department at hospital where delivered
- Bed rest will alleviate symptoms but not prevent a headache
- Record BP, temperature and pulse
- Paracetamol can be taken as necessary
- Dehydration should be avoided
- Caffeine might help
- Tell woman about possible diagnosis and that treatment is available
- Support with infant care
- Review as required

HEADACHES ASSOCIATED WITH HYPERTENSIVE DISORDERS

- If woman complains of headache and other symptoms of pre-eclampsia, urgent GP referral should be made
- BP ≥160/100 mmHg refer to GP urgently
- If woman has severe headache only and history of PIH, refer to GP
- Known hypertension—management as described, observe for symptoms of pre-eclampsia
- Review the next day in all cases
- Discuss hypertension with GP at any time if indicated

GENERAL ADVICE

- Avoid factors which precipitate or exacerbate headache
- Take short rest periods when possible during the day
- Do relaxation exercises to relieve tension

REFERENCES

Atterbury J L, Groome L J, Hoff C et al 1998 Clinical presentation of women readmitted with postpartum severe preeclampsia or eclampsia. JOGNN 27(2): 134–141

Barrett G 1996 Primary care for women: assessment and management of headache. J Nurse Midwif 41(2): 117–124

Berger C W, Crosby E T, Grodecki W 1998 North American survey of the management of dural puncture occurring during labour epidural analgesia. Can J Anaesth 45(2): 110–114

Broughton Pipkin F 1995 Fortnightly Review: The hypertensive disorders of pregnancy. BMJ 311: 609–613

Cesarini M, Torrielli R, Lahaye F et al 1990 Sprotte needle for intrathecal anaesthesia for Caesarean section: incidence of postdural puncture headache. Anaesthesia 45: 656–658

Choi A, Laurito C E, Cunningham F E 1996 Pharmacologic management of postdural puncture headache. Ann Pharmacol 30(7–8): 831–839

Cooper G 1999 Epidural blood patch. Editorial. Europ J Anaesth 16: 211–215

Crawford J S 1972 The prevention of headache consequent upon dural puncture. Br J Anaesth 44: 598–600

Crawford J S 1979 Experience with spinal analgesia in a British obstetric unit. Br J Anaesth 51: 531–535

Davey D D, MacGillivray I 1988 The classification of the hypertensive disorders of pregnancy. Am J Obstet Gynecol 158(4): 892–898

Department of Health 1996 Report on confidential enquiries into maternal deaths in the United Kingdom 1991–1993. HMSO, London

Department of Health 1998 Why mothers die. Report on confidential enquiries into maternal deaths in the United Kingdom 1994–1996. The Stationery Office, London

Douglas K A, Redman C W G 1994 Eclampsia in the United Kingdom. BMJ 309: 1359–1400

Duley L, Henderson-Smart D J 2000a Magnesium sulphate versus diazepam for eclampsia. Cochrane Review 3. The Cochrane Library, Oxford

Duley L, Henderson-Smart D J 2000b Magnesium sulphate versus phenytoin for eclampsia. Cochrane Review 3. The Cochrane Library, Oxford

Duley L, Gulmezoglu A M, Henderson-Smart D J 2000 Anticonvulsants for preeclampsia. Cochrane Review 3. The Cochrane Library, Oxford

Ferrazzani S, De Carolis S, Pomini F et al 1994 The duration of hypertension in the puerperium of preeclamptic women: relationship with renal impairment and week of delivery. Am J Obstet Gynecol 171(2): 506–512

Garcia J, Marchant S 1993 Back to normal? Postnatal health and illness. In: Robinson S, Tickner V Research and the midwife. Conference proceedings 1992. University of Manchester

Glazener C M A, Abdalla M, Stroud P et al 1995 Postnatal maternal morbidity: extent, causes, prevention and treatment. Br J Obstet Gynaecol 102: 282–297

Grove L H 1973 Backache, headache and bladder dysfunction after delivery. Br J Anaesth 45: 1147–1149

Gutsche B B 1990 Lumbar epidural analgesia in obstetrics: taps and patches. In: Reynolds F (ed) Epidural and spinal blockade in obstetrics. Baillière Tindall, London

Halpern S, Preston R 1994 Postdural puncture headache and spinal needle design. Metaanalyses. Anesthesiology 81: 1376–1383

Hopkinson J M, Samaan A K, Russell I F et al 1997 A comparative multicentre trial of spinal needles for Caesarean section. Anaesthesia 52(10): 1005–1011

International Headache Society Headache Classification Committee 1988 Classification and diagnostic criteria for headache disorders, cranial neuralgia and facial pain. Cephalagia suppl 7: 7–96

Katz J, Aidinis S J 1980 Current concepts review. Complications of spinal and epidural anesthesia. J Bone Joint Surg 62A(7): 1219–1222

Lamy C, Sharshar T, Mas J L 1996 Cerebralvascular diseases in pregnancy and puerperium. Rev Neurol (Paris) 152(6–7): 422–440

Linn F H H, Rinkel G J E, Algra A et al 1996 Incidence of subarachnoid haemorrhage—role of region, year, and rate of computed tomography: a meta-analysis. Stroke 27(14): 625–629

Lubarsky S L, Barton J R, Friedman S A et al 1994 Late postpartum eclampsia revisited. Obstet Gynecol 83(4): 502–505

Lybecker H, Djernes M, Schmidt J F 1995 Postdural puncture headache (PDPH): onset, duration, severity and associated symptoms. An analysis of 75 consecutive patients with PDPH. Acta Anaesthesiol Scand 39: 605–612

MacArthur C, Lewis M, Knox E G 1991 Health after childbirth. HMSO, London

MacArthur C, Lewis M, Knox E G 1993 Accidental dural puncture in obstetric patients and long term symptoms. BMJ 306: 883–885

McSwiney M, Phillips J 1995 Post dural puncture headache. Acta Anaesthesiol Scand 39: 990–995

Madej T H, Jackson I J B, Wheatley R G et al 1993 Assessing introduction of spinal anaesthesia for obstetric procedures. Quality in Health Care 2: 31–34

Magee L A, Ornstein M P, von Dadelszen P 1999 Management of hypertension in pregnancy. BMJ 318: 1332–1336

Pitt B 1973 'Maternity blues'. Br J Psychiatry 122: 431–433

Rasmussen B K 1993 Migraine and tension-type headache in a general population: precipitating factors, female hormones, sleep pattern and relation to lifestyle. Pain 53: 65–72

Saurel-Cubizolles M-J, Romito P, Lelong N et al 2000 Women's health after childbirth: a longitudinal study in France and Italy. Br J Obstet Gynaecol 107: 1202–1209

Shutt L E, Valentine S J, Wee M Y K et al 1992 Spinal anaesthesia for Caesarean section: comparison of 22 gauge and 25 gauge Whitacre needles with 26 gauge Quincke needles. Br J Anaesth 69: 589–594

Stein G S 1981 Headaches in the first postpartum week and their relationship to migraine. Headache 21: 201–205

Stein G, Morton J, Marsh A et al 1984 Headaches after childbirth. Acta Neurol Scand 69: 74–79

Stride P C, Cooper G M 1993 Dural taps revisited. Anaesthesia 48: 247–255

Sudlow C, Warlow C 2000 Epidural blood patching in the prevention and treatment of post dural puncture headache. Cochrane Review 3. The Cochrane Library, Oxford

Sztark F, Petitjean M E, Thicoipe M et al 1996 Subarachnoid haemorrhage caused by aneurysm rupture. Initial management of patients. Ann Fr Anesth Reanim 15(3): 322–327

Taivainen T, Pitkanen M, Trominen M et al 1993 Efficacy of epidural blood patch for post-dural puncture headache. Acta Anaesthesiol Scand 37: 702–705

Teunissen L L, Rinkel G J E, Algra A et al 1996 Risk factors for subarachnoid haemorrhage: a systematic review. Stroke 27(3): 544–549

Vandam L D, Dripps R D 1956 Long term follow up of patients who received 10 098 spinal anaesthetics. JAMA 161: 586–591

Van Gijn J 1997 Slip-ups in diagnosis of subarachnoid haemorrhage. Lancet 349: 1492

Walters B N J, Thompson M E, Lee A et al 1986 Blood pressure in the puerperium. Clinical Science 71(5): 589–594

Wasserberg J, Barlow P 1997 Lumbar puncture still has an important role in diagnosing sub-arachnoid haemorrhage. BMJ 315: 1598–1599

APPENDICES

Appendix 1

SEARCH STRATEGY

A comprehensive literature search was undertaken to inform each guideline. To ensure the accuracy and validity of the search strategy used, advice was given at various stages of the guideline development by systematic review experts from ARIF (the Aggressive Research Intelligence Facility), within the Department of Public Health and Epidemiology, University of Birmingham.

In addition to searching the bibliographic databases (listed below), the team also reviewed published guidelines and, in the absence of any primary research, relevant textbooks.

- Cochrane Library (Issue 1, 1999–Issue 3, 2000)
- MEDLINE (Ovid 1974–August 2000)
- BIDS
- CINAHL (Ovid, 1990–October 2000)
- MIDIRS (The Midwifery Research Database)
- Bandolier (via www)
- Embase (Ovid, 1990–October 2000)

Studies investigating the symptoms of interest during the postnatal period were first selected, and where such studies were absent or not of adequate quality, pregnancy related or general population studies were included. For each guideline the main focus of the search strategy was to identify studies relevant to community midwifery practice rather than hospital based care. Thus, for example, there is no reference in guideline 1 on Endometritis and abnormal blood loss to the evidence based management of primary postpartum haemorrhage. However, in the absence of community based studies in some cases the most appropriate reports from hospital based studies were included.

In addition to these sources, some references were obtained from World Wide Web guideline sites, for example the New Zealand Guidelines Group, and from hand searching of other specialist literature, for example newsletters of maternity organisations. This was important because studies of interest, particularly relating to midwifery or primary health care, may not have been indexed on an electronic database.

The original search list was sifted by one or more of the authors and inclusions/exclusions made on the basis of the study abstract and, where this was not available, the study title. Searches reflected the recognised hierarchy of evidence (see below). Initially, systematic reviews were identified, followed by randomised controlled trials, controlled studies and cohort studies. In those instances where none of these sources was available, examples of practice described in relevant textbooks were cited. Restriction to English language was applied at various stages of the search.

An example of the search strategy used to identify studies on the management of postnatal perineal trauma is given at the end of this Appendix. This strategy was used to identify studies recorded on Medline; similar strategies were used to identify literature for all of the symptoms of interest from the other bibliographic databases accessed.

References were included only if in English and published from 1950 onwards, although almost all are much more recent. Literature searches were first conducted between June 1996 and October 1997, then a second search was done between July 1999 and October 2000 to update the guidelines for publication following use in the IMPaCT study.

Hierarchy of evidence

A recognised 'hierarchy of evidence' was followed in searching and reviewing the literature. This is listed below and shows how standard study designs can be graded into a hierarchy of decreasing strength of evidence.

The best quality evidence comes from well designed randomised controlled trials (RCTs) or systematic reviews of RCTs. Next best are prospective studies with some form of non-randomised comparison group, or good cohort studies. The quality of evidence from this second

I	Well designed randomised controlled trials (RCTs)
II-1a	Well designed trials with pseudo randomisation
II-1b	Well designed controlled trials with no randomisation
II-2a	Well designed cohort (prospective study) with concurrent controls
II-2b	Well designed cohort (prospective study) with historical controls
II-2c	Well designed cohort (retrospective study) with concurrent controls
II-3	Well designed case control (retrospective study)
III	Large differences from comparisons between times and/or places with or without the intervention
IV	Opinions of respected authorities based upon clinical experience; descriptive studies and reports of Expert Committees.

(From NHS Centre for Reviews and Dissemination 1996)

level of studies is more variable, depending on sample size and ability to adjust for confounding factors. Retrospective studies with controls come next on the hierarchy, and studies with other forms of comparison follow these. Obviously the size, methodology and scientific rigour with which studies are carried out influence their strength as evidence, but this hierarchy will hold true as a basis for consideration of evidence.

There have been few randomised controlled trials undertaken within many of the postpartum health subject areas. Because of this, the trial team did not apply a scoring system to assess the face and content validity of included studies. Critical appraisal was undertaken of all included studies to identify factors which may have affected validity.

Example: search strategy for perinal pain

#1 perineal adj pain ti, ab	#14 13 and 5
#2 perineum/	#15 puerperal disorders/
#3 perineum. ti, ab	#16 puerperal infection/
#4 perineal. ti, ab	#17 or/15–16
#5 or/2–4	#18 5 and 17
#6 Exp pain/	#19 sutures/
#7 pain management/	#20 suture technique/
#8 pain postoperative/	#21 sutur$. ti, ab
#9 pain threshold/	#22 or/19–21
#10 'wounds and injuries'/	#23 5 and 22
#11 or/6–10	#24 dyspareunia
#12 5 and 11	#25 dyspareunia.ti, ab
#13 postnatal care/	

REFERENCES

NHS Centre for Reviews and Dissemination 1996 Undertaking systematic reviews of research effectiveness. CRD guidelines for those carrying art or commissioning reviews. University of York, no 4, p 33

Appendix 2

SYMPTOM CHECKLIST

I am going to ask if you have experienced any of the following health problems since having your baby. These are all health problems which many women experience after childbirth. If we know you have a particular problem, we may be able to offer advice or treatment to help it.

Since having your baby, have you experienced:

	Guideline No:	Date		Date	
		YES	NO	YES	NO
Abnormal bleeding	1				
Perineal pain or dyspareunia	2				
Abdominal wound problems	3				
Breastfeeding problems	4				
Urinary problems (ask about stress incontinence, UTI, voiding difficulties)	5				
Bowel problems (ask about constipation, haemorrhoids, loss of control)	6				
Depression	7				
Fatigue	8				
Backache	9				
Headache	10				

PLEASE REFER TO APPROPRIATE GUIDELINE FOR SUGGESTED MANAGEMENT OF EACH SYMPTOM IDENTIFIED

Appendix 3

USE OF THE EPDS

The guideline on Depression and Other Psychological Morbidity refers to the use of a screening instrument (the Edinburgh Postnatal Depression Scale, Cox et al 1987) for the detection of postnatal depression. The scale was administered to all women recruited to the trial by midwives using the new model of care on the twenty eighth day and at the 10–12 week consultation to screen for those at risk of depression. The midwives were not expected to initiate counselling or other treatment interventions, but to refer women who had high scores to their health visitor or GP for further assessment and management. Since there is concern that much psychological morbidity is unrecognised (Cooper & Murray 1998), it is important that efforts are made to ensure this is addressed, but discussion should take place to establish current practice in your area with regard to the identification and management of psychological morbidity.

It is important to ascertain if health visitors currently administer the scale to all postnatal women and, if so, when; and to ascertain what happens to women who have a high score. It is important to determine what current practice is in your area to ensure that the advice you give is relevant and that care is not duplicated. Please refer to the 'What to do' section for further advice on administering the EPDS.

REFERENCES

Cooper P J, Murray L 1998 Postnatal depression. Clinical review. BMJ 316: 1884–1886
Cox J L, Holden J M, Sagovsky R 1987 Detection of postnatal depression. Development of the 10-item Edinburgh Postnatal Depression Scale. Br J Psychiatry 150: 782–786

Page numbers in **bold** indicate figures and tables.

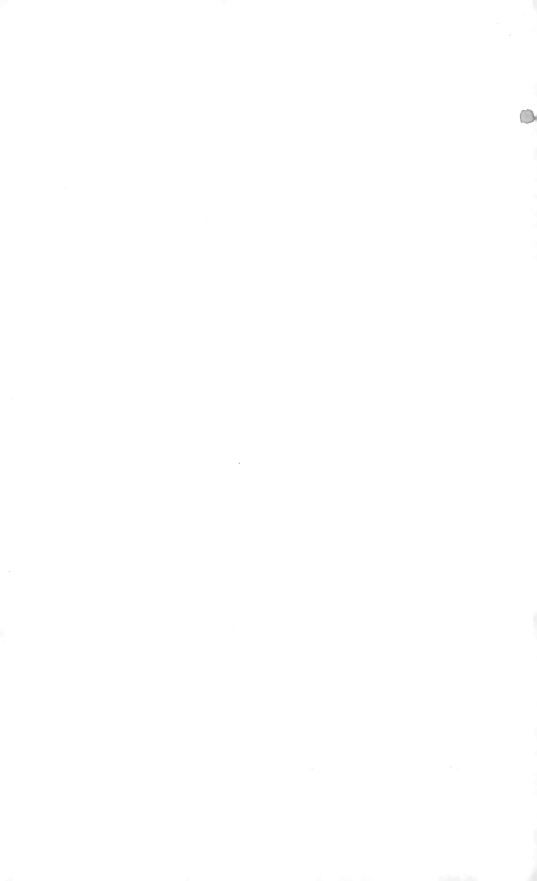